attrACTIVE WOMAN

attrACTIVE WOMAN

A Physical Fitness Approach to Emotional and Spiritual Well-Being

by

Marvel Harrison

Catharine Stewart-Roache

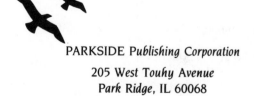

PARKSIDE *Publishing Corporation*

205 *West Touhy Avenue*
Park Ridge, IL 60068

Harrison, Marvel
Stewart-Roache, Catharine
  attrACTIVE WOMAN

ISBN   0-942421-07-8

Library of Congress   89-060259

Printed in the United States of America

10   9   8   7   6   5   4   3   2   1

DEDICATION

this book is dedicated to the
insightful, exciting, and playful
participants of the

NEW MEXICO WOMEN'S WELLNESS CONFERENCE

1984-1988

especially

FRANCES WOLFE

our friend and mentor
who continues to inspire us

Acknowledgments

During the late spring, summer, and fall of 1987, we ran through this book. We cycled it, swam it, canoed it, climbed it, walked it. As we did we talked about and shaped the book. But although we worked alone we were not alone. The spirits of our friends and mentors and women from the Women Inward Bound groups were very present to us and guided us in the process.

The following are some very special people we wish to thank for their talents, inspiration, and help:

Pat: encouragement in getting the computer and learning to use a word processor but especially for his continual interest in and enthusiasm for me and my active life-style.

Catharine

Jeffrey: for believing in me and this project from the onset, by encouraging me to experience my work, play, and feelings to their fullest.

Marvel

Paul: computer engineer who helped with "cosmic interferences" and midnight trips to Santa Fe.

Marvel's mother and sisters: all attrACTIVE women.

Participants of Women Inward Bound.

Dr. Liz-Beth Soybel, Dr. Glenn Chaffee, Lydia Pendly, Nancy Weaver, Judith Swarth and the Office of Health Promotion and Nutrition Bureau, Public Health Division, State of New Mexico.

Greg: illustrations and humour.

The following are more special people and places for which we are grateful; without them the book would not have come to be.

Grace, Iva, Ann, Art, Mary Jo, Marilyn, Dennis, Fairly, Curtis, Ginny, and Don; Santa Fe Baldy; Sandia Peak; Pajarito Mountain; Grand Tetons; Canadian Rockies; the Alps; La Luz Trail; Eastern Nepal; the Snake, Colorado, Yampa, Rio Grande and Salmon Rivers, Kirtland Air Force Base; Milford Track; Logan Canyon and Alamo Canyon, and Ghost Ranch.

Workshops and lectures:

Marvel Harrison and Catharine Stewart-Roache offer training seminars and educational programs about gaining emotional and spiritual well-being through physical activity. In addition, Marvel offers seminars for people with disordered eating and their families, and training for professionals. She also gives wellness workshops on nutrition, fitness, and stress management. Catharine leads workshops on being physical and spiritual, feminism, and physical activity after age forty.

For more information, write:

Marvel Harrison
1720 Calle Boca del Canon
Santa Barbara, CA 93101

Catharine Stewart-Roache
P.O. Box 8172
Albuquerque, NM 87198-8172

Contents

Foreword

Early in my personal growth, which I call "recovery," I recognized the need to develop spiritually, mentally, and emotionally. It took longer to learn to pay attention to my body. One of the first self-defeating coping behaviors I learned was to disown, or separate, *myself* from my body. I continued that process of separation even in recovery.

Many of us have disowned our bodies. Many of us did it to survive. But our bodies are as much *us* as our emotions, mind, and spirit. All parts are intertwined and will pay a price if we neglect one part.

My journey into physical self-awareness began when I learned to play. Learning to play didn't come easily, or naturally. It required commitment, focus, and a plan. My journey continued when I learned to dance. Next, I learned fifteen minutes of exercise in the morning could dispel mild depression and fear, and enhance creativity.

I delved more deeply into the wonders of the physical when I discovered the benefits of therapeutic massage. Memories and pain are stored in our bodies. Our bodies have messages for us. A body in shape can contribute to a well-tuned mind, open emotions, and a balanced spirit. And a little positive touch can counteract years of negative touch and energy.

Staying in touch with our bodies is essential to staying in touch with ourselves. Becoming physically active can help us discover and strengthen our sense of self, improve our capacity for intimacy and love, and bring into focus lessons we're struggling to learn other ways.

Loving our bodies helps us love ourselves—and others.

This book, *attrActive Woman,* came into my life at the right time. I had recently added swimming to my list of physical activities, and was blundering my way through a series of mistakes at the pool. I was swimming without goggles, without sealing and protecting my hair, and without warming up or cooling down. I was exiting the pool with red eyes, green hair, and stomach cramps. I didn't know why, and was about to give up, when this book explained what I needed to know.

attrActive Woman gently explores the importance of coming back home to live in our bodies, taking care of our bodies, and learning the lessons they have to teach us.

It also contains valuable tips on how to avoid green hair, red eyes, and stomach cramps if we swim, and tips on how to approach other forms of aerobic activities to gain maximum benefits.

I'm a novice at physical activity. This book helped me believe it was okay to be a novice, and okay to become active anyway. It offers welcome permission to accept, take care of, and love ourselves.

attrActive Woman is a common-sense approach to getting and keeping active physically. It's written in a way that makes a regular program of exercise manageable and appealing.

Melody Beattie

Introduction

Another book on fitness ! ! ! ! On aerobics? Aren't there
enough? Yes. And no. There are excellent books available that
give good solid information about what to do and how to do
it. There are good books about feeling good and dealing with
stress, with shifting gears when life calls for a change. There
are books for and about women. But we don't think there has
been one which explicitly links mental health for women
and a life style of being physically active in the same way as
attrACTIVE WOMAN.

Our belief is that as our bodies change, we are changed and
that we are never too old, or tired or busy to enjoy our bodies
and learn from them. We can learn lessons of strength—inner
and outer strength—lessons of self-discovery and persever-
ance. Through attrACTIVE WOMAN a woman can grow in
self-esteem; she can feel better about herself and herself IN
her surroundings. She can change and grow through physical
and psychological changes which she chooses herself, or which
she discovers on the journey inward.

Our emphasis is on using physical activity—play, sport, movement—as a basis of mental and emotional health. This is for
two reasons: this has been our experience, and this is being
scientifically proven.

My experience of depression in 1980 confused me because
all my old tools of dealing with being "down" weren't working
well. I had never felt so "down" for so long. I tried reading, praying, meditation, music. . . . I still felt very "down"
and helpless. A friend suggested I go swimming. I remembered

I used to like to swim when I was a young girl. But then I thought about going to the pool and how I'd look in a swim suit. This was adding to my feeling of "down". "Look," my friend said, "Why don't you take your fat thighs for a swim. They'd like it!." What did I have to lose? Only a bit of embarrassment.

My thighs liked it. I liked it. The feeling of movement; of cool water and cleansing; the refreshed sense of myself. I was slow; I had to stop a lot at first, but I was hooked. The depression lifted. Not because external conditions changed. They didn't. But I changed. I felt better about myself. I had more energy and confidence. When circumstances weren't moving, I was . . . in the pool. When life pressed me down, the water held me up.

Gradually, swimming became a part of my life. Later I learned about endorphines and swimmer's high. Physiologically there were reasons why I felt better, but there was a bit more. I had made a choice to do something. To act. To change. Not to accept feeling down . . . and out. A victim of my circumstances and feelings. More than endorphines was acting here. Growth and self-discovery were happening. Once in place, they were me on the move. Me becoming me.

Catharine

I have always been an active woman; I am fortunate to have been raised in a supportive and fun-loving family in a day and age when it was beginning to be acceptable for young women to be active. I enjoy white-water canoeing, hiking, skiing, and swimming. In short, I like to play. My regular activity is running. For years I ran without ever knowing why—nor feeling a need to justify it. I recall my Dad, who thrives on common sense, asking me, "Why do you simply run down the road? Why don't you run out to the barn and feed the horses?" I'd roll my eyes, sigh, and exclaim, "Oh, Dad, you just don't understand!" The reality was I didn't have an answer and I didn't understand, but I knew something kept me on the road.

Several years later after participating in a women's run, a reporter stopped me. She asked me the same old question: why do you run? I shrugged my shoulders, smiled, and told her it was so I could enjoy all the fun things in life. She quizzed me. "You mean, you don't have any fun running?"

"No it isn't that. I do enjoy running, but it's much more than the actual 'pounding the pavement.' Somehow it really is, well, fulfilling." The reporter frowned, shook her head, and walked away. Obviously, I still didn't understand why I was running down the road. This incident spurred me to contemplate the question further. I learned my running time was very sacred to me. I enjoyed endless creative ideas and did lots of professional and personal planning and decision making; occasionally it was a sharing time with friends. More often it was personal time to feel, think, and get to know myself. My running was a powerful energizer for me . . . emotionally and physically.

Through the years I've come to know running as "active meditation," a time for me to get to know Marvel. But I never realized the power running held in my life until I was devastated by a broken relationship. I was shattered emotionally by the loss of a love, my playmate, and friend. It felt like my entire world had crumbled around me. I was numb, unable to concentrate, and it felt like the pain would never end. Fortunately, I had the road to pound on. Even though emotionally I was paralyzed and my innermost spirit felt strangled, I was still physically capable of moving. Running was familiar. It helped relieve the pain I was living. It became a place for me to work through my emotional rawness. I felt the pain of my anger, hurt, fear. I owned them and let go of them as I ran . . . I was moving. Now I was beginning to understand why I was "running down the road."

Marvel

These are our stories. Other people, other countries are discovering that being active—being physical—is important to life and a healthy spirit. Australians are familiar with "Life: Be in it." In Canada they use the word "participACTION."

Our ideas and experiences aren't all new. Many books have been written about fitness, but somehow the division between body and mind remains. Muscles are built . . . but a stronger self is referenced in another book. We will bridge the gaps between body, mind, and spirit. We will write about women in a whole and, perhaps, holy way.

Originally we designed the attrACTIVE WOMAN program for women over forty because we felt that they had been left out of much that is associated with sports and physical activity. Complaints poured in: "Women over forty aren't the only ones who need to reclaim their bodies; they aren't the only ones dealing with 'downs' and divorces." We gave in. The women were right. Being attrACTIVE is important at any age.

Our interest is in women like ourselves who have grown up in societies just a little uncomfortable with women's bodies. Societies unused to recognizing bodies as sources of wisdom and mental health—more used to working separately on the physical, then perhaps the mental or emotional. Our aim is to see the interconnectedness of ourselves and live with a consciousness of how very much we are one being, one self, one person.

The format for attrACTIVE WOMAN is an eight-week group of not more than ten women who meet once a week to process their experience of the physical at an aerobic level. We assist them in selecting an activity which suits their needs and interests, give them information about principles of physical and emotional health, and discuss how to listen to their bodies and apply the wisdom available through them to their daily living. We are excited when we see a decrease in depression and an increase in confidence and self-esteem because their bodies have grown stronger and more fit. At the same time, we recognize that many women are unable to commit to our program held on certain days in certain locations. So we have written this book as an alternative way for women to get involved in our program of emotional, physical, and spiritual health. We intend for this book to be a work book, to be something which women not only read, but move through. Movement is the focus. Movement for women of all ages, sizes, spirits.

Often we begin our programs showing George Sheehan's film "Coping with Life on the Run." We will conclude this introduction by quoting him:

> Given the choice, most of us would give up the reality of today for the memory of yesterday. . . . or the fantasy of tomorrow. . . . But for the active in mind and heart and body, the child and the poet, the saint and the athlete, the time is always now. They are eternally present.

"Now" is a healthy and holy place to be. To play. To love. To live. We invite you to begin with us an experience of attrACTIVE women—women inward bound.

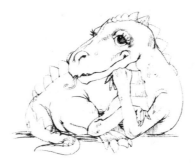

Dragon Notes

There are different ways of looking at dragons. To medieval people they were powerful, commanding, and terrifying creatures. St. George was sought to find them and run them through with his lance. But another legend, of more ancient origins, appeals to us. This is the legend of Martha (to some, Margaret) who lived in southern France (or Italy, or Switzerland) long, long ago. She is depicted in iconography as a mature woman exuding confidence and victory who has conquered the dragon, but without violence. The stories vary. In some she is more clever than the dragon, in others she reasons with her and the dragon agrees not to terrify the people any longer, and in still others she blesses the beast. One image shows Martha walking into a town with the dragon following meekly behind her.

Her? Yes, legend has it that all dragons were female. We have thought about dragons and thought about women who have varying "dragons" inside themselves who threaten their very lives unless they are tamed. Self-destructive dragons of depression, anxiety, dieting, overwork and expectations, ignorance, low self-esteem and even self-hate. These dragons need frequent taming—they don't need to be treated violently. Like Martha, we can approach them with wit and charm. And as they are tamed, we can incorporate their strength and power. Instead of "damsels in distress" we can become capable women who are no longer victims of these dragons.

With this book we are adding to the legend. We believe that this taming of dragons has resulted in the dragon's conversion to Martha's goodness; she will assist us in illustrating exercises and good practices of attrACTIVE women of any age. We find her charming and hope you fall under her particular spell also.

Psychology of Being AttrACTIVE

*A man once said to me, "I don't mind you telling
me my faults, they're stale, but don't tell me my
virtues. When you tell me what I could be it
terrifies me." I was surprised then, I understand
now, because I believe we may be faced by the need
of living our strengths.*

Florida Scott-Maxwell

When it comes to a physical image, the past few decades
(hundreds of years?) have been confusing for women. Society
has dictated that we must be feminine and has shown us how
in many different scenes: passive, girdled, slim-as-Twiggy, skirts
up to our thighs—down to our ankles, burning bras, sitting on
Supreme Courts, working on construction sites, getting di-
vorced, managing alone, flirting, demanding, pleading, thinking . . . changing. We are bombarded with images of what we
should or could look like ("before" and "after" . . . as if the
"before" were not also precious, and me), and how to be "sexy"
(there is real confusion here). Articles and books abound which
deal with women's problems on the job, at home, and in the
world at large.

To be a woman today is very demanding. It requires more
than just thought or know-how drawn from our foremothers
or contemporary gurus. Clearly we must find our own selves
and believe in ourselves; we must be able to move about in
relation to others. Often we ask friends or relatives about how
to live. We read books, we seek spiritual guides. Seldom do we
include our bodies in this search for life's wisdom. Even more
rarely do we look to our bodies as sources of wisdom and guides
for living. Amazingly our bodies can be sources of wisdom and

self-knowledge. In a symbolic, metaphorical way our bodies in motion can be sending us powerful messages. Messages of hope, strength, power. Messages of *basta* (enough).

This is what makes attrACTIVE WOMAN unique among fitness programs and books. Throughout the development of your activity (your play, your sport) a consciousness is emphasized: What am I learning here which I can (or perhaps need to) incorporate into my daily living?

A few examples may help.

CATHARINE I have already mentioned my aerobic exercise beginning with swimming; mentioned that I felt better and kept up with my program because of that. But something else happened. Something happened in my psyche, in my image of me. A personality change? Probably not completely, but surely a modification. Taking that hour for myself four times a week said:

> "You are special; worth some time set aside." Goodness knows with five kids I had "set aside" a lot of time for others; as a counselor and minister I had "set aside" many hours for people who I thought were important—even if *they* weren't so sure.
>
> "You are supported." Water held me up when I swam and that feeling was important to me at that time of my life.
>
> "You can dump all sorts of worries and burdens and confusions in the water and leave cleansed and refreshed from the pool."
>
> "You are beautiful and weightless in the water. Utterly graceful. You are free of burdens for this hour." When I would go home, or back to work, that feeling would linger and peace would be mine.
>
> "There is a silent world for you." Before swimming I was unaware of how much I needed a bit of silence in my day.
>
> "You can be in charge of this hour and your activity in this hour." Now that is a great feeling for a mother and a terrific feeling for someone "on call" privately and professionally.
>
> "You are one strong woman." I could see how I had progressed. I could go farther and faster than last week or last year.

With these kinds of continual messages I began to believe in myself more. It felt good. My list of swimming messages could go on. They are my list. Each one of us will have different learning experiences. One thing I know for sure: What I learned by moving in the water was learned very differently and took root in me more strongly than had I learned them through other methods. Books, tapes, conversations, magazine articles—none of them were as thorough a teacher as my own body—once I began to pay attention to it, trust it, and reflect upon my experience.

The confidence I gained through swimming led me to consider other physical activities as part of my problem solving when my life situation got very difficult. In 1983 one of our children became mentally ill. The process of diagnosis was long and difficult. There was almost unbelievable strain on each one in the family, on my marriage, and on myself. I knew the effect swimming had had on my life. Now I began to wonder if an increase in aerobic activity from three or four times a week to five or six times might be helpful. I was concerned that increasing my swimming might lead me to burn out on swimming, and it was too special to be put in such jeopardy. To make a long story short, I got a bicycle. My symbolic thinking went something like this: If life is such an uphill climb, maybe if I actually learn to climb hills I can get some help, I can make some changes so each day doesn't seem so difficult.

This proved to be true. It took quite a bit of time and self-discipline, but the payoff was very great. From my bike and my body I learned that I couldn't try to climb hills in the same gear as riding flat terrain. When my life had been "flat" (or at least "flatter") I could go through it in high gear with many "teeth" (translate: many commitments and activities), but when it was difficult and "uphill" I needed to drop back into an easier way of moving forward, I needed to shift down into a lower gear, a gear with less tension; I learned to ride through my daily living more smoothly with fewer activites and causes. It didn't make all my days easy and all my decisions easy, but it made life possible. I *was* able to function. I honestly believe that if I had stayed in my "high gear" approach to the hills in my life at that time, I would not have gotten through, or I would have been sick, or perhaps have gained 50 pounds, since overeating is one of my less healthy ways of coping with stress.

MARVEL It has only been recently that I have recognized many of the insightful things I have been learning from my body all the years I have been active. It is not that I hadn't been learning anything in the past, it is just that the learning was such a natural part of the benefits of being active, I was not truly conscious of the tremendous opportunity for emotional and psychological growth. When I have spent time reflecting about what I have learned from being an active woman, it has been almost as invigorating as the activities themselves! It is truly a joy to share a few examples . . . greatest of all perhaps is the sense of accepting challenges.

I remember one Sunday morning bicycling with some friends on what I had been informed was going to be a leisurely morning ride, followed by brunch. Wrong—it was a rigorous thirty mile ride of roller coaster ups and downs and one hellish hill. My friend Lo and I were lagging behind the rest of the group and had been enjoying some great conversation (in between my gasps for oxygen!) about building careers and the possibility of my opening a private practice in eating disorders counseling. I had been sharing with her how anxious I was to take on such a challenge and how afraid I was about failing at the endeavor. On the last hill, a seemingly endless climb, she half shouted to me, "If you can make it up this hill, my dear friend, you can do anything!" And yes, I made it to the top of the hill, only with great concentration, intense effort, and support from my companions. I since endured the struggles and triumphs of the new phase of my career with the same concentration, effort, and support I learned on that "hellish hill"!

A couple of years later this same wonderful woman and I were enjoying an afternoon of reminiscing when I shared my "temptation" to write this book, again revealing my fears and anxieties about such a challenge. She simply smiled, squeezed my hand, and whispered earnestly, "Don't you remember the hill?" I truly am grateful for my body, which can teach me so much, and my insightful friend Lo.

I learned many years ago, on the road while running, that when I push too hard, too fast, or don't pace myself, it's no fun. It feels too much like work. Regardless of whether my endeavors are personal or professional, this phenomenon holds true. Life is too short not to "know joy" so I am attempting to apply what I have learned on the road to my everyday life. The really exciting part for me is that the road, the hills, and the rapids are still out there with an abundance of untapped re-sources for me (through my active body) to learn from!

• • •

These are our very personal psychological insights. Some might be applicable to you, others may not ring a bell at all. But from our experiences and observations of other women's lives we have come up with four characteristics we think women need in order to meet today's challenges of change, survival, and growth and we have seen how our bodies can be involved in this necessary and exciting endeavor.

WE NEED TO KNOW OURSELVES

We need to find out about our unique "stuff"—the qualities that are a gift of life first of all to ourselves, and then to others. By seriously exploring physical activity, a woman can learn something about her uniqueness and specialness. For example, we can learn if we are women of endurance who can be counted on in the long run figuratively or literally, or if we're ones who are quick and dynamic . . . catalysts who can get ourselves off to good starts and finishes.

Through our swimming, canoeing, running, and cycling, we both have discovered that we are women of endurance. We have learned to pace ourselves for the long run . . . we needed to learn this in order to live a bit better. Often each of us would

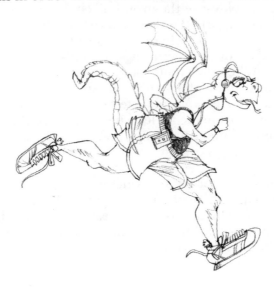

try to burst into a situation and finish fast when we hadn't learned the skills, or weren't suited for that style in the first place.

We found out how to be more efficient in our endurance; to find a pace at which we can go a long, long way and then stick to it, even if others pass us by. In the long run, "my pace is right for me." (And we often pass up the ones who were off in a flash but faded too soon.)

We're talking about what we've learned in living life from doing our activities. Not from reading alone, but from listening to our bodies and trusting them . . . trusting them to know ourselves as unique individuals. After all, we've been with our bodies a long time. For years each of us tried to find out about ourselves from going to school, reading, and listening to others. These are all good and necessary, but it took a long time to realize that our bodies could be trusted and were wise.

Of course, we've had help along the way—"no (woman) is an island"; there are women and men who can help us pay attention to our body-wisdom, just as they too have learned from their own and others' experiences.

CATHARINE This was certainly my experience when I was on trek in Nepal. Trekking in Nepal is hard work and it is not like hiking in the U.S. I watched how the sherpas and porters walked up those steep, steep hills and I watched our guide. He and I were the oldest of the group. Each day we would see the 20-year-olds dash off. "Find your own pace; not anyone else's pace. Find that tempo where you can just go and go; if you push yourself, you will be tired too soon—today, and on the whole trek." When the going got particularly rough and I knew he and I were going about the same speed, I'd move up close behind (and usually *below* in a steep area) and put my foot in his footsteps. This helped a lot when I was tired. It was better than him giving me a hand up. I was still the one doing the work, and I had discovered a way to help myself, through another.

As I thought about my trekking at night I thought about it in relation to my whole life. I wasn't just walking in the eastern foothills of the Himalayas, I was learning to live better. My Nepali body was teaching me: pace yourself and you will be able to endure. Listen to others who have walked a similar path, they have wisdom too. My three weeks in such a different country and terrain demanded that I learn to receive, accept from others, accept from life. Something that I as a "professional" giver (chaplain, counselor) needed to learn better. Balance. Good mental health is about balance. What better place to learn balance than with Buddhist sherpas, on steep ascents and descents. What better teacher than my body!

• • •

WE NEED STRENGTH . . . INSIDE OURSELVES

By increasing physical strength we symbolize to ourselves that we can change an image of weakness or inadequacy to one of strength and capability. Through a program of regular aerobic and anaerobic level activity women not only build stronger muscles, but stronger psyches.

Day by day an active woman sees real physical change and because of this she can more easily believe in herself as one capable of change and growth. She can come to know herself as someone strong enough for the job, the challenges, the pressures and stresses of life.

As one discovers new muscles one can be discovering new strengths. An unused muscle quickly tells us, "I haven't done that before (or in a long time)." Likewise, when we try new things or experience new emotions, we often feel inadequate—weak in the face of it. Just as with our bodies, so it is with our emotions and minds. They become stronger when they are used—and not abused. Slowly stretching our muscles prepares our bodies for more activity so that they can become stronger. Slowly venturing into new facets of ourselves, new feelings and thoughts, adds to our flexibility and makes psychological strength not only possible but probable. And the same caution applies: learn to use, not abuse. Too much too soon, with no preparation, tears at ourselves, just as it tears up our bodies. This is particularly challenging in our society of "If a little is good, more must be better." This attitude ignores quality or even pits it against quantity—as if one is more important than another.

MARVEL Sometimes I can go many miles and the quantity feels good—a sense of accomplishment is tied up in that; other times, how many miles I have gone doesn't tell the tale. When

I was on a canoeing expedition in the Canadian wilderness, there were long, hard days of paddling loaded boats 50 to 60 miles and there were even longer and harder days of portaging those loaded boats only three-quarters of a mile . . . miles told very little about what the experience was! I learned another fascinating lesson from the river concerning the question of quantity. I learned to kayak in Idaho where there are big, high-volume, roaring waters like the Salmon and Snake Rivers. To "run" these waters the elements of force and velocity are required to "punch through the rapids" and maintain an upright position on the other end! Later, when I kayaked in Europe I quickly learned I had little opportunity to employ my skills learned on the whitewaters of Idaho. Now I was faced with very rocky, shallow, and extremely technical water where force and velocity put one at high risk of destroying body and/or boat. The techniques now required included precise, quick movements, slowing the boat down by back paddling to allow time to assess the next maneuver and finesse the next rock or hole. Very simply I learned the necessity of judging apparently similar, yet very different situations where it was critical to use opposite techniques. The rivers' personalities have spoken to me and taught me. Their wisdom guides me in working with people. Taking some time out to understand some of their differences and learning new skills has been a great advantage to me.

• • •

To become a stronger woman, experience your body as it grows stronger; it can teach you much about how you uniquely approach growth and change. It can tell you if you are one who needs a slow steady increase in trying something new or if you are someone who can move along rather rapidly into new ventures. Pretty useful information for us to discover—not outside of our experience, not in another's textbook, but here "at home" in our body-self as attrACTIVE WOMEN.

Women today also need to feel strong in relation to others. We need to know that we can't be pushed around. The price of believing that others have all the power and control over our lives is a high one indeed. Women around the world are realizing that they are not property, that they are valuable workers, valuable human beings. Slowly and swiftly, women are demanding equal rights, equal opportunities in this challenge called living.

If I Can Run a Mile

In day-to-day living we can enjoy and use this newly discovered strength. If I know myself as someone who can walk ten miles, lift 75 pounds, ride 50 miles, swim a mile etc., I am much less likely to be intimidated by telephone solicitors or high pressure sales persons of any sort. When a woman allows herself to become physically strong, that strength can be a foundation for psychological strength. "I can run the mile on my own" can translate into "I can talk to the boss . . . write the proposal, take a trip on my own, run the program . . . write a book." I am much more likely to hold my ground (hold on to my opinions) with boss, employees, family, friends. From a position of self-strength (confidence) I am much more able to listen, and perhaps even change my ideas because I *choose,* not because I am overwhelmed or cowed.

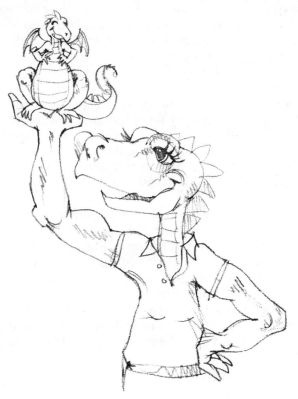

WE NEED TO KNOW OUR LIMITATIONS

Women are not made up only of strengths. A truly wise woman knows her limits and her weaknesses; she must learn this so that she can take care of herself and so that she can focus on, and build upon her strengths.

Most of us have watched some athletic competitions—at least a bit of the Olympics. What strikes us is that these athletes have had to find out not only at what they excel, but also what they don't do so well. They don't pick the latter. So often we act because someone says "please do this or that," or we try things that are expected of us when we aren't good at them at all. No athlete would get talked into an event which she knew was her weakness. She has learned this by paying close attention to her body in motion.

Listen to Your Body

As you go through the attrACTIVE WOMAN program you will be urged many times to "listen to what your body is telling you." When it tells you about weakness it's telling you something very important. When we recognize and accept our weaknesses we learn how to choose goals and challenges that don't defeat us. We can select small steps that build our self-confidence and self-trust in our professional or personal lives.

When faced with physical or psychological limitations or weaknesses, various courses of action are possible. For example, I can make note and simply try something else, easier or more enjoyable, where success is more likely. Or, I can approach the situation differently and perhaps get different results. Or I can decide that this is something that I want to try anyway and perhaps gain some additional strength in what was formerly a weakness.

Just facing a limitation causes me to consider what my goals and values are, and that is very important in a mentally healthy life. I ask myself, "Is this idea or feeling something which is very important to me? Or is it unimportant in the long run? Do I want to spend a lot of energy—a lot of me—on it? Or is it better to go on to something else?"

Time and again we find ourselves and others willing to spend 85 percent effort on a problem which, if we only thought about it—if we considered our limitations—we would wisely only spend about 10 percent of our energy.

I do not have an unlimited bank account of life-energy. I must choose many times a day. Knowing my limitations allows me to spend wisely. Past experience is a very good teacher. Specifically, past experience of my body's limitations is a good teacher.

WE NEED SELF-ESTEEM

Perhaps self-esteem is just the result of knowing ourselves, as strong, capable women who are not Wonder Woman, but women with limitations who learn to love and accept their limitations and strengths as part of their unique makeup. Perhaps it is self-esteem which allows us to move through life with heads held high, able to face a few surprises and still hold steady on a course.

Sometimes trying to get a clear definition of self-esteem is not so easy. We read about self-esteem and we listen to those whom we counsel, and it is obvious when it is not present in someone. Abraham Maslow defines self-esteem as need for respect, for confidence based on good opinions of others, admiration, self-confidence, self-worth, self-acceptance. Physical activity is not the only means of achieving or supporting self-esteem but it is an *immediate* source, and one readily available (rather inexpensive, too). Built into being physically active are most of these characteristics. Have you ever known anyone to have a low opinion of someone because they swim, walk, hike, cycle, etc.? Of course not! In this society (thank God, unlike Victorian society) women who are active are admired. Day by day the messages of my attrACTIVE self are:

I am worth time and attention.

I am grounded in my body; I accept it, and am not at war with it.

I am moving (not stagnant), flexible (not rigid).

I am energized for living.

Perhaps all of this boils down to self-esteem as the ground of good mental health—as the primary need of women today. In religious circles a few years back there was a popular slogan: God doesn't make junk. We believe that if you give your body a chance, you'll find out that it isn't a piece of junk. It is a resource, a source of wisdom, and can help you lead a more mentally healthy life.

The Battle With the Body

The trouble is many of us women have histories of battles with our bodies. Some of us are scared of them or hate them, or, we have put in years criticizing them and finding fault. In this war-like atmosphere (which the media and we ourselves have created) it comes as no surprise that it is difficult—nearly impossible—to trust our bodies enough to listen for the wise messages. But the messages are there.

One of the consequences of the "battle of the bulge" has been that being overweight, overfat, or obese can lead to a decision not to be active "because I'm just too fat." In their enthusiasm to get people to shed excess fat, writers in the field of fitness have focused on goals of low percentages of body fat and body weight. Perhaps the definitions of obesity for women as "more than 30 percent body fat" or "greater than 20 percent of ideal body weight" are accurate *physiologically,* but we have seen this "fact" used in such a way that women have damaged themselves *psychologically.* This number (given by somebody else) borders for some on obsession. It becomes the focus of psychological energy. The quality of life itself then becomes measured by these numbers. "I am being bad (good)"; "It's a good day (bad day)." We think that this can be a dangerous amount of power given to these thoughts. Self-esteem gets associated with percentage of body fat and body weight! Many have decided that if they weigh more than a certain amount or have a greater percentage of body fat, then they shouldn't or couldn't be active. An exciting group in New York City has done much to counter this. Greater Women of New York is a fitness group for overweight, overfat women who *move.* They feel better; they have more positive images of themselves. Wisely, they have medical consultants who check out their aerobic programs to insure that they are safe for larger women, but they are not being told, "If you are overfat, don't move—don't enjoy your body." Physical aerobic activity is not a "for slims only" proposition. Of course, some common sense is needed. A gradual increase in activity is important. Monitoring heart rates is a necessity. But so it is for all of us.

CATHARINE If I had believed that overfat women (or ones with fat thighs) shouldn't get serious about athletics, I never would have gotten in that swimming pool. What a loss that would have been!

• • •

Physical Activity and Emotional Well-Being

Current scientific research is proving that our bodies are sending important messages to our brains and selves. There is an increasing body of literature in Canada and the United States which supports this link between emotional well-being and physical activity.

At the University of New Mexico, Dr. Dennis Lobstein and his associates report that participants in their study were able to decrease depression. Their joggers exhibited lower perceived stress, lower physical malfunctioning, decreased anxiety, and decreased hostility; they were more emotionally stable. It is important to note that these participants were not clinically diagnosed as depressive; they were folks like you and us who get "down," very "blue," who have bad days when they "can't get started." Lobstein et al. (and others at Cornell University) have shown that an aerobic level of activity helps alleviate these problems.

Today, scientists are qualifying and quantifying the relationship between stress and disease as well as the positive effect of regular exercise on reducing stress and promoting physical and mental health. Cardiologists have been observing this link for some years now and prescribing regular aerobic exercise as commonplace treatment for many patients. They respect the interconnectedness of the mental and physical in their patients. A heart is not only an organ, it is a symbol of life and how one lives. High anxiety, deep depression, etc., are physically as well as mentally unhealthy.

When one is active at an aerobic level more oxygen gets to our brain and chemicals are produced which are mood altering. Adrenalines and endorphines are real physical entities, which make a difference in how one feels. We might say they are "natural drugs" which can enable us to feel happier, energized and just plain good. It is only fair to mention that research is showing that exercise can be abused, too. Overexertion can tear down our bodies, fatigue our minds. Runner's "high" can lead to an imbalanced runner's addiction . . . not just the positive addiction about which Dr. Kenneth Cooper writes so convincingly. The key is still listening to and respecting the messages our bodies send to us. People need to ask themselves, "Am I controlling my exercise, or is it controlling me? Am I using exercise to avoid problems?"

The point is that, as in all aspects of life and health, there is no one remedy which can disregard balance and thought. Good physical health through an active body is, generally speaking, a fine path to good mental health. It can also be a complement to individual or group psychotherapy.

It is the purpose of the attrACTIVE WOMAN program to develop (or heal) a relationship between self and body. There is so much to be gained if we allow this psychological door to open.

We are one creation: body, mind, spirit, emotions. The ancient Hebrew word "basar" conveys this idea of unity. The health of one affects the health of the other. The truly total woman: AWARE, ACTIVE, ALIVE.

Recommended Reading

Women and Self-Esteem, Linda Tschirhart Sanford, Mary Ellen Donovan. Penguin Books, New York, 1985.
The Aerobic Program for Total Well-Being, Kenneth H. Cooper. Bantam Books, New York, 1982.

2

Getting Physical

Sociologists tell us play has meaning without purpose. We must learn to play. Far too many fitness routines are packed with purpose but devoid of meaning. You've made it through when your activity brings both meaning and purpose.

Gordon W. Stewart

Everyone knows regular exercise is "good for us" and there are many reasons why. Sometimes those reasons seem too much like someone else's and we are uncomfortable with them . . . or they don't seem to suit us. Only you can identify your own very meaningful and personal reasons for getting and staying active. Among the goals for participating in an activity program, there are some which are psycho/social in nature, for example:

- improved self-image, confidence, self-esteem
- less depression and mood swings
- less anxiety
- increased ability to deal with everyday stressors
- greater confidence in personal and professional life
- an overall sense of well-being
- personal time
- social time
- greater personal energy
- increased spiritual life
- clearer thinking; alertness

Some are more obviously physical but have psychological, symbolic, or metaphorical implications:

- stronger bones and muscles (a sense of a stronger *me*)
- attractive, trimmer, and fit body ("trim" down my life)
- better coordination and flexibility (getting myself "together"; becoming more flexible with myself and others)
- healthier sleep patterns (accepting rest as life-giving; greater ability to "let go")
- fewer physical complaints of aches, pains, and constipation (developing a more positive attitude)
- stronger heart and lungs (stronger "heart," increase in "spirit" or "breath of life," a more "airy" attitude)
- greater endurance (not "giving up" so readily)
- competition (learning that I don't perform at peak level all the time, learning that others' excellence can "bring out the best" in me—learning not to be threatened by others, enjoying success, dealing with failure—as part of the whole picture of life)

Obviously our list could go on and on. One goal sometimes cited is "to live longer." We have purposely excluded it because we are not interested in the arguments about whether or not a person's life span increases with regular activity. Our interests lie not in the quantity of life but in the improved quality of the life we are living now . . . living life to the fullest as attrACTIVE women.

MARVEL Nearly every time I give a personal fitness presentation, I get challenged on the topic of "What about that guy Jim Fixx who died of a heart attack when he was running? I don't want to end up like him . . . dead in my tracks." I gently respond with "Do you know how many hundreds of people on that same day suffered a cardiac arrest while watching T.V.? Sleeping? Eating?" Usually the challenger smiles and backs off and I comment about the odds not being in favor of the "couch potato."

• • •

Only you can decide what your reasons for regular aerobic level activity are and what your personal goals will be. Be sure the reasons and goals are for you . . . not your friend, spouse, or companion. Don't try to impress someone. Just yourself. It is important to sort through your reasons and to not begin simply because "I know I *should* exercise." Sound familiar? All those "shoulds": I should take time for the kids, I should eat this or that, I should get more sleep, I should drink more water. It's not nice to "should" on people . . . especially yourself! It is a persistent self put-down and a person spends so much time and energy "should"ing that nothing gets done.

PHYSIOLOGICAL REASONS FOR REGULAR EXERCISE

Let getting rid of the "exercise should" be the first step in your program of healthy thinking and feeling good. Chapter 3 will consider how to set your goals and move toward them; here we will detail the physiological reasons for regular sustained—we hope fun—activity. The general categories of goals are improved physical, mental, and emotional well-being. Aim for any one area and chances are you will pleasantly surprise yourself with increased health in another area as well!

A Stronger Heart and Cardiovascular System

To strengthen your heart and cardiovascular system you must give your heart a workout. Your heart is a muscle about the size of your fist. You need to work this muscle in order to strengthen it, just as you would work other body muscles to increase their strength. The stronger your heart (your pump) is, the fewer times it has to beat to keep your system functioning well. You will learn more about a stronger heart in the section on aerobics later in this chapter.

Stronger Bones and Muscles

Strong, thick bones are less likely to break. It is that simple. As we age our bones have a normal tendency to become weaker and thinner. Besides growing older (about which none of us has a choice), there are other factors which hasten the bone-thinning process, like cigarette smoking, being inactive, and not consuming enough dietary calcium. To begin with, our bones are generally thinner than our male counterparts. This bone thinning, in its disease form, osteoporosis, is a serious health problem, particularly for women, because it puts a person at high risk for breaking bones.

A broken bone may have serious medical complications due to prolonged bed rest (i.e., increased blood clots, pneumonia, bed sores). In addition, the psychological stress on a person who has lost independence (and perhaps self-worth) due to being immobilized by a major bone fracture, can be devastating. At best you're unhappy and not feeling "like myself."

When bones are exercised they become thicker, stronger, and have sufficient blood estrogen, provided a person is consuming enough dietary calcium. Women need about 1,000 milligrams of dietary calcium per day to sustain healthy bone thickness. Following menopause, the requirements increase to around 1,200 milligrams (for more about calcium in our daily diet, see chapter 4 and appendix D).

As well as strong bones we need stronger muscles to help prevent minor aches and pains—particularly in our lower backs (. . . sound familiar?). In order to strengthen a muscle you must contract it and regularly give it a workout. This does not mean developing bulging muscles! Women can have strong muscles without them being large and bulky since it is the hormone testosterone (much more present in males) which is necessary for significant muscle enlargement. We have also heard women grumble their concern that if they are active and build muscle, then stop exercising, "all those big muscles will turn to fat." Impossible. Muscles cannot turn into fat (one less thing to worry about). Although fat cannot turn into muscle either, what does happen is that through exercise, muscles will tone and tighten your body into an attractive, strong, working, available-to-do-what-I-want home for *you*.

Flexibility and Coordination

Better flexibility helps prevent injuries by decreasing the amount of tension exerted on the muscles. The more flexible you are, the less likely you will be to pull or tear a muscle because your muscles will be able to stretch further. Coordination is improved when movements and motions are repeated and muscles are strengthened and become more flexible. Being more coordinated and flexible opens up a whole new world of activities which you thought you might never have tried, and your daily movements will reflect a more graceful and confident you.

Once we remember hearing a physical therapist lecture on caring for the body. She discussed the concept of treating each of our body joints like a hinge of a door. If you were to open the door the full distance once each day it would not suddenly be rusted and stuck shut. It is when you leave them unused that your joints will seize up and not work for you; remember to give each joint a full round of motion each day. Becoming more flexible reduces muscle soreness and is done through slow, deliberate, and gentle stretching (see pages 32-41).

AttrACTIVE, Trim, and Fit Body

We hope you noticed that losing weight was not given as a reason for exercise. It was purposefully omitted because it is so much healthier to change your body composition than to simply lose body weight. When you lose body weight, what are you losing? Water, fat, muscle tissue?!? When you lose fat tissue and increase your lean tissue, so altering your body composition, you may or may not lose body weight but you will be trimmer, more toned, and wear smaller clothing sizes. This is accomplished through being active in an aerobic activity program and not by dieting. We have much more to share with you on the whole concept of dieting and how women are "dying to be thin" (see chapter 4).

Muscle tissue weighs about 25 percent more than fat tissue. It takes up much less space and actually burns more calories on a constant basis—fat is bulkier and uses very few calories and sits around keeping us warm. You are better off wearing an extra sweater!

Body composition is, most simply put, the measure of how much of your body is lean muscle and how much is fat tissue. It is a better measure of health and fitness than body weight is. There are many ways of predicting composition including:

- skin fold calipers (the pinch test)
- electrical impedence machine (simple electrode hook-up)
- body circumference measurements (tape measure)
- hydrostatic weighing (weighing under water in a large tank)

There is no "perfect" method for measuring your percent of body fat—short of dissecting a cadaver! Presently, much research is being conducted in this area of exercise physiology. To date the method most used in research is the hydrostatic weighing. But it is important to realize there can be many variations in the results of measurements being taken and it would be wise to use the measurement as a guideline of change rather than expecting a particular number to be exactly right for you. We don't want to see percentage of body fat becoming the oppressor which bathroom scales have been in the past! Neither indicates self-worth and both are flawed as meaningful data points. There are tremendous differences reported in percentages of body fat taken on the same person by competent exercise physiologists. (We have read reports of 12 percent variations on the same person: one physiologist measured 18 percent, another 30 percent!)

CATHARINE Years ago I had my percent body fat determined with skin calipers. The result was 31 percent. Recently I wondered how much my percent of body fat had been reduced since my accelerated cycling program of the past three years. (I had cycled about 9,000 miles, averaging about 80 to 120 miles per week during the season.) So I had another qualified exercise physiologist take my measurements. (MISTAKE. Always use the same method and same person for this kind of testing.) She calculated 39 percent! This could have been a real bummer. I could have believed her figures and not my own body. I chose not to. I know my percent of body fat has not increased. I can look in the mirror; I can feel myself in my clothes. But so often women don't trust themselves. They will trust data in magazines, or from professionals. The findings at this point in time are not accurate enough and the techniques for measurement are not controlled enough to warrant that kind of trust. Usually women know when they carry around too much fat. (I know I do carry more than I need—but I also know it has not increased in the past three years.)

• • •

If you are still interested in being measured call a Registered Dietitian or hospital, university exercise physiology department, or fitness center to check for credentials and services offered.

Facing the Fats

If you want some help in "facing the fats" there are several simple self-administered "tests" which can give you an idea of whether you have any fat to lose.

- Mirror Test—Look at yourself naked in front of a full length mirror. Is anything "rolling" over or bulging out? Where is fat deposited?
- Bust/Waist Comparison—Compare your waist measurement with your bust measurement. Is your waist smaller?

- Pinch It Gently Test—This easy test is to give you an idea of where your fat is "hanging on." Much fat is located right under the skin and to find it you will need a friend's assistance. Hold your right arm out in front of you with your palm held open and upward. With your left index finger and thumb, gently pinch the skin on the back of your arm halfway between your elbow and shoulder. Be sure and pull the skin away from the muscle so you only have skin and fat in your pinch. Have your friend measure the distance between your thumb and finger. How much can you pinch? More than an inch?
- Spare Tire Pinch—Find your waist by tying a string around your middle where you would comfortably wear a waistband of a skirt or pants. Stand up straight and with your index finger and thumb, gently pinch the skin on your side about one to two inches above the string. Measure the distance between your thumb and finger and see how much you can pinch. More than an inch?

Most women have an idea of whether they are overfat or underfat without taking any tests. If you have "faced the fats" in one way or another it would be a healthy decision to begin a graduated aerobic activities program. We are also concerned about women who appear slim externally yet are overfat internally; they run many of the same physical health risks as their obviously overweight, overfat sisters. Of even greater concern are women who are underweight and underfat due to the self-destructive behaviors of dieting, purging, laxatives, pills, or poor nutrition. Both these groups of women would also benefit from entering a graduated aerobic activity program.

OK. Hang on, women, you are about to embark on an inward- and outward-bound adventure. You are on your way to becoming truly attrACTIVE. And remember: You're Worth It!!

Getting Started

PAR-Q and You (Developed by the British Columbia Ministry of Health) There is a simple way to begin this experience and it makes sense to boot! Begin by filling in this self-administered questionnaire known as the PAR-Q—a Physical Activities Readiness Questionnaire for adults. This handy tool is a screening device which will assist in isolating the small number of adults who are not able to participate in physical activity or need a more thorough evaluation prior to beginning. Most women will be cleared through the PAR-Q immediately—so give it a try:

- Take your time.
- Follow the instructions.
- Read it thoroughly.
- Answer each question thoughtfully.
- Read and follow the advice which applies to you.

PHYSICAL ACTIVITY READINESS QUESTIONNAIRE (PAR-Q)

A self-administered questionnaire for adults, PAR-Q is designed to help you help yourself. Many health benefits are associated with regular exercise, and the completion of PAR-Q is a sensible first step to take if you are planning to increase the amount of physical activity in your life.

For most people physical activity should not pose any problem or hazard. PAR-Q has been designed to identify the small number of adults for whom physical activity might be inappropriate or those who should have medical advice concerning the type of activity most suitable for them.

Common sense is your best guide in answering these few questions. Please read them carefully and check the YES or NO opposite the question if it applies to you.

YES	NO	
_____	_____	1. Has your doctor ever said you have heart trouble?
_____	_____	2. Do you ever have pains in your heart and chest?
_____	_____	3. Do you ever feel faint or have spells of severe dizziness?
_____	_____	4. Has a doctor ever said your blood pressure was too high?
_____	_____	5. Has your doctor ever told you that you have a bone or joint problem such as arthritis that has been aggravated by exercise, or might be made worse with exercise?

_____ _____ 6. Is there a good physical reason not mentioned here why you should not follow an activity program even if you wanted to?

_____ _____ 7. Are you over age 65 and not accustomed to vigorous exercise?

If You Answered Yes to One or More Questions

If you have not recently done so, consult with your personal physician by telephone or in person BEFORE increasing your physical activity and/or taking a fitness test. Tell him/her what questions you answered YES on PAR-Q, or show him/her your copy.

After medical evaluation, seek advice from your physician as to your suitability for:

- unrestricted physical activity, on a gradually increasing basis.
- restricted or supervised activity to meet your specific needs, at least on an initial basis. Check in your community for special programs or services.

If You Answered No to All Questions

If you answered PAR-Q accurately, you have reasonable assurance of your present suitability for:

- A GRADUATED EXERCISE PROGRAM—A gradual increase in proper exercise promotes good fitness development while minimizing or eliminating discomfort.
- AN EXERCISE TEST—Simple tests of fitness (such as the Canadian Home Fitness Test) or more complex types may be undertaken if you so desire.

Postpone Activity

If you have a temporary minor illness, such as a common cold.

The PAR-Q advice to "postpone" if you have a temporary minor illness, such as a common cold needs to be taken seriously. On very rare occasions an otherwise healthy person who has a fever may experience a heart problem during vigorous exercise like running activity. It is best to start your activity when you and your body are ready to be active. Listen to your body, get to know your body, and if you are ill, chances are your body is requesting a mini vacation. There will be times during your new active life-style that your body will want a break. So do it a favor and give it one!

Types of Activities

Since you've decided to join the ranks of attrACTIVE women we will explore many of the possibilities of pursuing your new found life-style. Let's begin with a quick review of the many activities a person can enjoy while becoming physically and emotionally fit. Generally, there are four categories of activities or exercises including:

Flexibility exercises like yoga, stretching, and dance all enhance your balance, improve posture, reduce joint discomfort and lower back pain, and offer an opportunity for peaceful relaxation. Stretching also plays an important role in injury prevention (see pages 32-41).

Strengthening exercises include lifting weights (both free weights and utilizing machines) and calisthenics. Developing strength is necessary for performing daily tasks independently with ease and comfort and it can improve your posture. This kind of activity is not aerobic.

Skill Building exercises include most of the recreational activities people enjoy such as: downhill skiing, bowling, golfing, horseback riding, softball, and football (playing it, not watching it!). Most games and team sports are anaerobic activity because of their start and stop nature. They are especially important for developing coordination, balance, and offer many of us, young and old alike, some wonderful social experiences besides just being a lot of fun!

Aerobic exercises are essential for development of a strong, healthy heart, and cardiovascular system. They will help strengthen bones and improve your endurance. With aerobic activity the fat levels in your blood change. For example, the beneficial high-density lipoproteins (HDL) increase and the total cholesterol decreases so there is a lowered risk of arteriosclerosis or hardening of the arteries. Aerobic activities help us burn more stored fat for fuel and therefore are the basis of developing a lean, trim, and streamlined body.

Some of the best activities for aerobic conditioning are:

- cross-country skiing
- square dancing, tap dancing
- swimming
- jogging or running
- brisk indoor or outdoor cycling
- brisk walking or water walking
- aerobic dance classes

Other activities which provide a desired conditioning effect if done with enough intensity include:

- dancing
- racquet sports like squash, tennis, racquetball, or handball (a person needs to be fairly skilled at these sports to enjoy them at an aerobic level)
- roller skating or ice skating
- horseback riding (for the horse only!)

The most efficient exercises for fat loss are the aerobic activities listed above. However, in order to feel your best and for great pleasure, enjoy a combination of flexibility, strengthening, anaerobic, and aerobic activities. We are going to elaborate on the areas of activity which we believe truly can lead you to an overall sense of well-being and balance. Your attrACTIVE WOMAN program will target aerobic activities and in addition will encourage stretching activity as part of your warm-up and cool-down time.

AEROBIC ACTIVITY AND THE FITTNESS FORMULA

People often ask "what makes an activity aerobic?" There is a simple formula to follow so you can calculate what in your life-style is aerobic. It is the FITTness formula: To get the most from an aerobic activity it must have all the components of the formula. The FITT part of FITTness is an acronym for the following:

> F is for FREQUENCY or "How often?"
> I is for INTENSITY or "How hard?"
> T is for TIME or "How long?"
> T is for TYPE or "What activity?"

Let's look at each of these important components of FITTness separately.

Frequency—How Often?

Fitness, like sleep, cannot be stored—five hours of activity on the weekend does not take care of your body's needs for the week. Thus, a regular activity program is necessary if you are to reach and maintain a healthy level of fitness. A program of three to five days per week is optimal for most women. Two rules of thumb to follow are:

• aim for being aerobic every other day, and
• avoid missing exercise for more than two days in a row.

Intensity—How Hard?

There is a pace at which activity is vigorous enough to condition the muscles and cardiovascular system, yet not overly strenuous. This pace is called the *target* or *training heart rate* and is often referred to simply as the talk/sing test. That is, if you can't talk comfortably while active, then you're working too hard. If you are able to sing while active, you're not working enough.

The Target Heart Rate is somewhere between 65 to 80 percent of an individual's maximum heart rate (MHR). If you have not been doing aerobic activity at least three days per week for a few months, aim for your *starting target heart rate*. This pace will elevate your heart rate to 60 to 70 percent of your maximum—high enough for fitness and fat loss benefits, but not so high that you become exhausted or risk injury. Actually, some studies indicate greater fitness benefits at 65 percent MHR than when working over 80 percent.

To determine your Starting Target Heart Rate, use the chart below. First, find your age in the chart. Your Starting Target Heart Rate is the corresponding number in the middle column. This is how hard your heart has to be beating so you and your heart are getting a healthy workout.

As you progress in your aerobic exercise program, aim for your *keeping fit target heart rate*. This number is in the last column, across from your age.

Your Target Heart Rate is based on taking your pulse during your workout for 10 seconds *immediately* after stopping your exercise. Ten seconds is long enough to be accurate and short enough to approximate your pulse rate at the time of stopping. If you are 37, you are aiming for a 10-second Starting Target Heart Rate of around 21 or a Keeping Fit Target Heart Rate of 24. If you are 58, you are aiming for 16 as your Starting Target Heart Rate or 21 as your Keeping Fit Target Heart Rate.

Note: Check your heart rate after the first five minutes of activity, at the peak of your workout and as you cool down. Continue your activity for several minutes. *Don't ever just stop immediately, because your heart rate needs to go down slowly.*

TARGET HEART RATE
(10 Second Count)

AGE	STARTING TARGET HEART RATE*	KEEPING FIT TARGET HEART RATE**
10-14	21-24	26-28
15-16	21-24	25-27
17-18	20-23	25-27
19-21	20-23	25-27
22-24	20-23	24-26
25-27	19-23	24-26
28-30	19-22	23-25
31-33	19-22	23-25
34-36	18-22	23-25
37-39	18-21	22-24
40-42	18-21	22-24
43-45	18-20	21-23
46-48	17-20	21-23
49-51	17-20	21-23
52-54	17-19	20-22
55-57	16-19	20-22
58-60	16-19	20-21
61-63	16-18	20-21
64-66	15-18	20-21
67-69	15-18	19-20
70-72	15-17	18-19
73+	15-17	18-19

*60%-70% Maximum Heart Rate
**75%-80% Maximum Heart Rate

First of all find your pulse. Everyone *has* a pulse. Some find it a bit tricky to locate. Patience and persistence will enable you to find it, we guarantee. The most convenient places to get a pulse are at the wrist (radial pulse) or the neck (carotid pulse).

To get your wrist pulse, turn your wrist so that the underside is up (and all the veins are showing). Place the fingers of your other hand so that your middle finger is pressing down on the wrist—slightly over the center towards your thumb side. Don't try to get your pulse with your thumb, as thumbs have their own pulse.

Now count the beats while your watch ticks off seconds (a second hand or a digital watch will work). In a 10-second period, how many beats? This chart will tell you what is a proper number of beats in a 10-second period for your Starting and Keeping Fit Target Heart Rates in your age group.

The carotid artery can be felt on either side of the neck about an inch back of the adam's apple. When pressing the carotid artery, use the right hand for the right side of the neck and the left hand for the left side. This practice will help you avoid pressing too hard on your throat with your thumb and causing dizziness or actually lowering your pulse.

The diagrams below show the location of the carotid and radial arteries and the proper technique for taking your pulse. Remember your Target Heart Rate is only a general guide. Your Target Heart Rate is based on taking your pulse for 10 seconds immediately after stopping your exercise momentarily. To take your pulse, gently press the carotid artery or the radial artery with the index and middle fingers for 10 seconds.

The Target Heart Rate is not etched in stone; it is only a

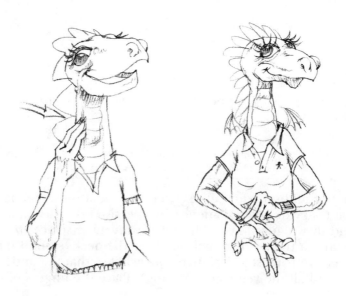

general guide. If you're a couple of beats either side of the target rate and it feels good, that intensity level is right for you. Experiment and find the right pace for you. After a while, you'll have a natural feel for the appropriate level of activity and be more familiar with your active body.

Before you get started with your activity program, before you are in the middle of walking or running, practice taking your pulses. Relax in a chair where it is quiet and you can really notice what's going on in your body. Locate either your radial or carotid pulse and position your fingers correctly. Then take your pulse for 10 seconds. Of course, after activity your pulse will be faster than at rest. Do not be discouraged if it is a struggle to locate your pulse—it will be easier when you are active, and besides, you can use the talk/sing test if necessary.

One reason behind all of the pulse monitoring is to measure how strong your heart is getting. A stronger heart means it has to beat fewer times and your body uses oxygen more efficiently to do the same amount of daily work.

Over a period of time, say six to eight weeks, your resting pulse rate can drop maybe two points. All this planning and work for a two beat drop? Big deal!

It really *is* a big deal. A few simple calculations show us that two beats per minute equals 120 beats per hour which equals 2,880 beats per day, or 20,160 beats per week, which is a significant 1,048,320 beats in a year. You're a millionaire! It is not uncommon for women to lower their resting pulse from 85 to 65 beats per minute—this is a total savings of over 10 million beats per year. In short, an investment in aerobic training means a great cardiovascular saving. So the idea is to give your heart a workout by *increasing* your heart rate for a short time (20 minutes) at an aerobic level several times a week. After a period of a few weeks (six to eight weeks) of regular aerobic workouts, your resting heart rate (heart rate taken before you get up in the morning) will decrease and your heart will be working less.

CATHARINE Mine dropped 20 to 25 beats the first summer I got serious about bicycling. I hadn't been concerned about a rapid pulse. I was "within range" at 90. But I can tell you I feel a lot better with it in the 60s. (Not everyone will experience this exact change.)

• • •

Time—How long?

The basic rule on length of time for aerobic exercise in order to gain cardiovascular fitness is to be active at your Target Heart Rate for a minimum of 20 minutes. We recommend after you've started a graduated program, make a minimum of a 30 minute commitment—5 minutes to warm-up, 20 minutes at your Target Heart Rate and 5 minutes to cool down. Now there are many reasons to be active longer than 30 minutes. For instance, the longer you stay at your Target Heart Rate, the more stored fat tissue your body will be using for energy and you will be losing body fat. Longer activity will also develop your endurance. Besides, maybe, just maybe, you will enjoy having an active body and will want to do it more. Beyond the minimum time for good health you will discover your comfort zone for the length of time for you to be active. Above all enjoy yourself— if you are really pushing to add a few minutes, give your body a break—build up time slowly.

Type—What Activity?

We get endless questions on "what type of activity counts as aerobic?" The answer is simply an activity which:

- is continuous and steady
- has rhythm—without stopping and starting
- uses the largest muscle groups (legs and buttocks—yes, those are **muscles** back there!)
- can be done by a healthy person for a minimum of 20 minutes

So, if an activity such as brisk walking, tap dancing, cycling, running, etc., meets these criteria, it is aerobic!

PHASES OF AEROBIC ACTIVITY

There are three major phases to being aerobically active:

1. Warm-up
2. Aerobic activity
3. Cool-down

It is necessary to incorporate all three phases into your regular program in order to get the full benefit of the activity and to prevent injury.

Warm-up

The warm-up phase (5 to 15 minutes) prepares your body for action! It consists of both gentle stretching and light activity. The purpose is to slightly accelerate the heart rate, warm up the muscles of the back and extremities, and to stretch tight connective tissue at the ends of the muscles. This process is lubricating the inner parts of your body so functioning is smoother and easier and you can do more activity before discomfort occurs. It is a must for injury prevention. Keep in mind these exercise guidelines as you perform this series:

- The exercises are gentle movement type or stretch-and-hold style. **There is no room for bouncing or jerking.** Think about and repeat in your mind over and over: Gentle, slow, easy movement.

- NO PAIN PERMITTED!! "I don't do pain!" The old myth of "no pain, no gain" is hogwash. Pain means something is not going right; you are overstretching or overworking your muscles and chances are you are doing more harm than good. If you experience pain during any phase of your program, go easier for awhile and if the pain continues, seek professional medical advice. Remember: NO PAIN means MORE GAIN.

- *For people presently receiving professional care for back problems or any other medical concerns,* follow only those exercises and activities outlined for you by your physician or physical therapist.

- *Keep breathing!* There is a natural tendency to hold your breath while doing many exercises. Think about inhaling and exhaling rhythmically on each repetition and keep breathing normally while holding and relaxing into the stretch. Exhale whenever you bend, twist or exert effort. If you find it difficult to keep a rhythm of breathing, count out loud as you follow the series, this will force a regular breathing pattern.

- Begin with five repetitions of each exercise. Hold each stretch position for five seconds initially. As you progress stay in the hold position for one or two seconds longer until you have reached 12 to 15 second "holds."

Following is a series of simple exercises appropriate for both your warm-up and cool-down phases of activity. Choose several from the list and remember the guidelines apply to all of them.

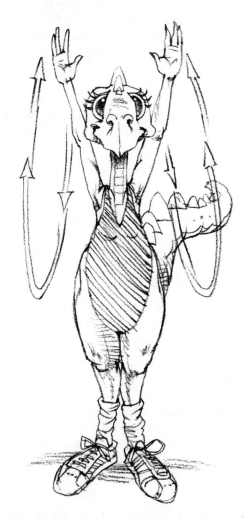

Arm Circles—Complete slow, full, sweeping circles with one arm and then the other. Forward, then backward. Next repeat with both arms. Exhale each time arms come down.

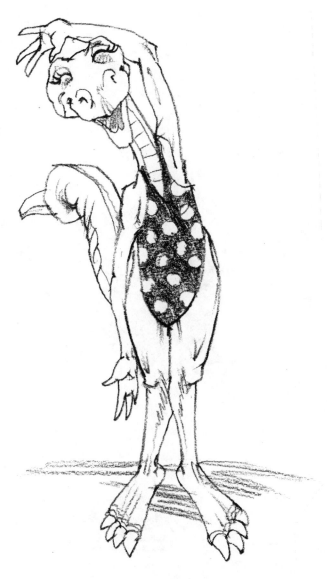

Side and Overhead Stretch—Place one arm overhead, reach down the side of the leg with the other arm while exhaling. Hold. No bouncing. Alternate to other side and repeat.

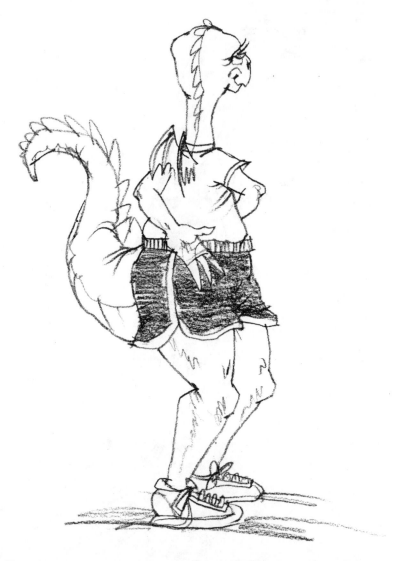

Trunk Twists—Place hands on hips, bend knees slightly, twist trunk slowly in one direction while exhaling. Hold. No jerky motions. Alternate to other side and repeat.

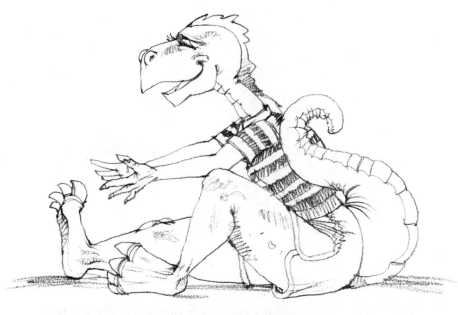

Sit-Stretch—Sit with one leg straight and one leg bent, with the sole of the bent leg's foot near the knee of the straight leg. Gently curl upper body toward knee of straight leg and with hands reach forward while exhaling. Hold the stretched position. No bouncing. Relax, then repeat. Alternate leg positions and repeat.

35

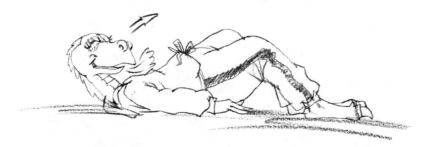

Peek-Ups—Lie on back with knees bent and place feet flat on floor. Keep back on the floor, lift head and shoulders and look toward knees. Exhale, relax, and repeat.

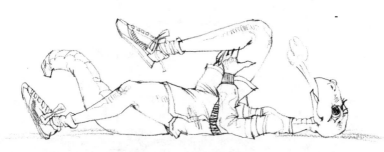

Single Knee Press—Lie on back with one knee slightly bent. Grasp hands behind other knee and bring knee toward chest while exhaling. Hold. Relax. Alternate with other leg and repeat.

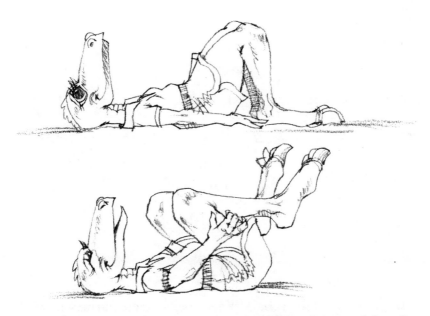

Double Knee Press—Lie on back, both knees bent and feet flat on floor. Grasping hands on back of thighs, gently pull knees toward chest while exhaling. Hold. Relax. Repeat.

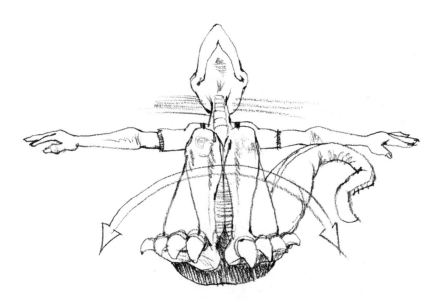

Hip-Twister—Lie on back, knees bent, stretch arms outward at shoulder level, keep back of head touching floor. Pull knees gently toward chest, then roll legs to one side toward floor while exhaling. Alternate to other side and repeat.

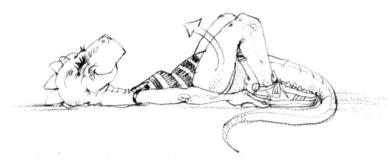

Pelvic Tilt—Lie on your back with knees bent. Press your lower back to the floor while rotating pelvis forward and exhale. Relax. Repeat. (Often recommended in your daily routine if you have lower back problems; check with your physician.)

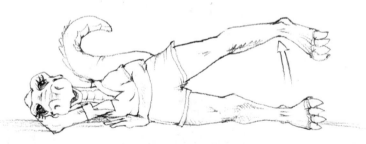

Side Leg Raises—Lie on one side with head resting on forearm. With toe pointed toward floor, keep top leg slightly bent and raise it slowly while exhaling. Hold. Lower leg slowly. Repeat. Same on other side.

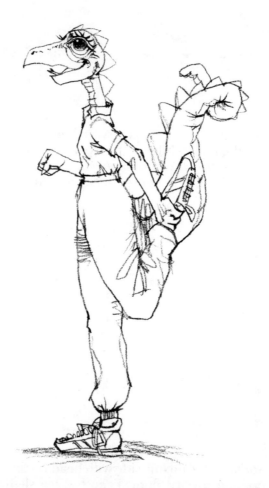

Thigh Stretch—Stand with legs shoulder width apart. Bend one knee, grasp the foot from behind and pull gently toward seat. Hold. Relax. Repeat. Alternate with other leg. It is sometimes recommended to use the right hand grasping the left leg and vice versa. Balance yourself by holding a chair if necessary.

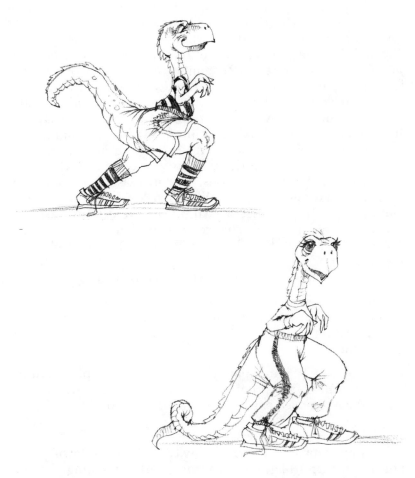

Gastroc Stretch—(*Gastroc* refers to the calf muscle.) Place one foot in front of the other with toes pointed forward. Front leg bent and rear straight. Gently rock forward over front leg to stretch rear calf muscle. Keep heel of rear leg flat on floor. Hold. No Bouncing. Repeat. Alternate leg positions.

Soleus Stretch—(*Soleus* is the flatter muscle below the calf and above the ankle.) Hands on hips, right foot eight inches in front of left, feet flat on floor. Keep upper body erect, bend both legs and stretch the muscles below the calf of the back leg. Hold. Change legs. Repeat.

Aerobic Activity Phase

The aerobic phase is truly the "heart" of your activity. In this phase you can experience spiritual, emotional, and physical growth. This is where you take yourself out on the road or down to the pool and find out what you are really made of.

Now is the time to take your selected aerobic activity and put it into your lifestyle. Remember a minimum of three to four times per week is required. Build your week around these dates with yourself. The key will be to begin gradually and slowly. In appendix A we have outlined programs for each of the aerobic activities: walking, running, cycling, swimming, and cross-country skiing—from start-up through healthy maintenance levels. Do Not Overdo It! Many women start out by trying to do too much. In doing this, you increase the chances of hurting yourself and you will be much less likely to continue your activity. Treat your body kindly and gently and ease into activity so you have the chance to experience all that being attrACTIVE has to offer. The keys will be to begin sensibly and to persist.

Should you develop uncomfortable signs such as:

- chest pain
- undue shortness of breath
- palpitations
- dizziness . . .

STOP the activity immediately! Check with your physician before continuing. Fortunately only a very small number of healthy women ever experience any of these problems.

Cool-Down Phase

An important end to your activity is the cool-down phase. This is a return to light activity and gentle stretching. Cooling down helps prevent dizziness or light headedness, muscle cramps, or other injuries. It is one more opportunity to be good to your body.

Take a minimum of five minutes for this phase. Simply keep moving at a slow enough pace so your heart rate declines gradually. Whatever your aerobic activity is, do it at a much slower rate. For example, if you were cycling, ride slowly or walk your bicycle, or if you were walking briskly, amble along slowly for five minutes. In order to help slow you down and relax, take in some deep breaths and exhale slowly and deliberately. Keep moving slowly for five minutes. Whew! What a wonderful sense of well-being!

A Note on Injuries

By following the above three phases of your activity program you will most probably enjoy injury-free activity. **In the event of any injury do not try to exercise through it.** The majority of injuries occur when a person is rushing through the phases, neglecting to warm-up or cool-down, or pushing too hard. It really is easy to get excited about this new life-style and the temptation to overdo it will be there for most of us. Resist this temptation by knowing your body will need time to catch up with your mind. Remember a major part of the attrACTIVE WOMAN experience is to bring body, mind, and soul a little closer. Not overdoing it will be one of your first challenges.

In case of a minor injury, immediate action can keep your recovery time to a minimum. The most common musculoskeletal problems are sprains and strains. Muscles and tendons suffer strains generally from overuse, and not warming up or stretching appropriately. Sprains occur at the joints and generally involve the ligaments. For example, if a cyclist is unprepared and overexerts herself, she may suffer a sprained ligament in the knee.

The simplest, most straightforward treatment of these injuries is to follow the **R.I.C.E.** formula:

Rest is essential to allow adequate recovery time. Returning to your activity too soon will set you back reinjured. Your activity may resume as mobility and pain allow.

Ice is best applied immediately. Never just hold ice on an area. "Massage" the area until the ice cube melts, or put a cloth between the cold substance and the injured area. Icing needs to be done for about 15 to 20 minutes at a time. For more serious injuries like a strained calf muscle you would be wise to ice it every three to four hours for the first two days.

Compression is simply pressure applied to prevent swelling. Wrap the injured area tightly but comfortably with a bandage wrap (such as "ACE") and leave it on overnight. Be sure not to wrap it so tightly as to cut off blood circulation. (It is best to check with your physician.)

Elevation aids in reducing blood flow to the injury by allowing the edema to "drain" due to gravity. Keep the injured area up as much as possible for the first day or two.

The sooner you initiate treatment by the R.I.C.E. formula, the better. Minor injuries will respond favorably and quickly. Any more serious problems will require some professional medical advice.

Obviously, like anything else, the key is prevention. Follow the steps outlined earlier in this chapter to prevent minor aches, pains, strains, or sprains!

CHOOSING THE ACTIVITY THAT SUITS THE attrACTIVE YOU

Now that you know what an aerobic activity is, which is the best suited activity for you? There are two basic guidelines:

- The activity needs to meet the aerobic criteria of the FITT-ness formula.
- It must be, above all, something that you enjoy and interests you enough to motivate you to continue for an indefinite period of time—hopefully a lifetime!

You do not have to "love" the activity or have it as a "positive addiction" but if you detest it, chances are you won't hang in there doing it for very long. Consider what is convenient for you and feasible in your daily schedule. If you have been inactive, have joint problems, or are overfat, activities like swimming, walking, or cycling will be more gentle on your joints than running. Brisk walking is an activity that more people keep as a lifetime habit than any other activity. It is convenient, simple, safe, inexpensive, and can be done alone or with others. Overall it is very feasible and healthy.

Consider the following questions and then make a decision about which activity to try first.

- Do I want to do my activity solo or with a friend(s)?
- How accessible do I need the activity to be? (i.e., is the swimming pool close to my home or work?)
- Do I need an activity which I can take with me when I travel?
- Do I have any physical limitations, such as joint problems or asthma, which need special consideration? (See our note on programs for differently abled people in chapter 3.)

- Do I want some excitement and challenge with my new plan? (exotic goals, competition, new identity, travel)
- What do the weather and safety conditions dictate in my area?
- Am I a person who needs a "touch of class" in my life? Does a commitment to a formal class sound like a good idea for getting started or continuing my program?

Seldom is any one activity just right for any of us. Possibly a combination of activities is more your style. Hiking might be a weekend option, while walking at lunch might be right during your work week. There is really no particular time of day to exercise that is healthier than any other time. If you live for "cuddling under the covers" in the morning—a program that starts at daybreak will most likely be a dismal failure. People report lots of positives for any time of day: "First thing in the morning and I feel great all day." "A noon hour activity keeps me from having a down time in the middle of the afternoon." "Running right after work gives me a peaceful transition time between work and home." Through experimentation you, too, will find your "magic time" that fits the attrACTIVE you.

Some people find joining a class works for them. Spas, YWCAs, city or county recreation centers, etc., offer an endless array of activity-class options. In choosing your class, use the following evaluation tool to select a safe, sound aerobic program.

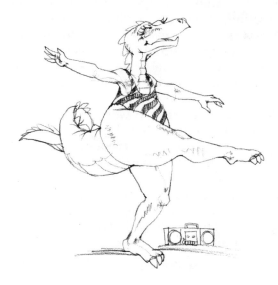

CHECKLIST FOR A SOUND AEROBIC CLASS

Answer the following questions yes or no:

____ 1. Is a personal health history form such as the PAR-Q and/or medical release form required for your participation in the aerobic activity?

____ 2. Are aerobic training principles such as the FITT formula explained and then followed during the class?

F — Frequency is three to five times a week, alternate days recommended.

I — Intensity of 60 percent to 80 percent of maximum heart rate (target zone).

T—Time is 20 to 30 minutes in target heart rate zone.

T—Type of activity—aerobic, slow, continuous, rhythmic, uses largest muscles.

____ 3. Are individual Target Heart Rate zones explained, established, and monitored regularly?

____ 4. Is the emphasis of the class on aerobic activity and good "heart health" rather than movement, dance technique, or getting "skinny quick"?

____ 5. Does the class allow for a warm-up phase (5 to 15 minutes), aerobic phase (20 to 30 minutes), and cool-down phase (5 to 15 minutes)?

____ 6. Is gentle, slow, easy stretching included in the warm-up and cool-down phases of the workout?

____ 7. Is your instructor aware when students are overworking, i.e., above Target Heart Rate zones, profuse sweating, irregular breathing, or red faces?

____ 8. Are variations of each exercise demonstrated so people of different fitness levels may participate?

____ 9. Are outside aerobic activities encouraged or similar classes offered if your class meets less than three times per week?

____ 10. Do you have a sense of well-being and/or satisfaction when you complete the class?

____ 11. Are your instructor's credentials and professional preparation acceptable? Professionally prepared instructors will have a background in fitness, injury prevention, exercise technique, planning, anatomy and physiology, teaching methodology, and will have attended training sessions specific to aerobic activity instruction.

If your evaluation concluded with 11 answers "yes," you have found a safe place to be attrACTIVE. ENJOY!

After making an activity selection it is unrealistic to expect to meet instant joy, but it need not be a dreaded bore. The right activity for you will suit your size, shape, personality, and life-style. Your activity will become a part of *you* . . . renewed, very alive.

A Quick Review

As a summary of this chapter, here is a 10-point checklist for you to follow while initiating your course of action:

1. ___ Think about what your reasons for being active are and write them down.
2. ___ Take the PAR-Q. Follow the instructions carefully.
3. ___ Consider assessing your body composition and if you meet the criteria, take the fitness level test(s). This self-testing is optional.
4. ___ Choose the aerobic activity which will best suit your size, shape, personality, life-style, pocketbook and— most importantly—that is fun!
5. ___ Make taking care of yourself a priority. You are worth it.
6. ___ Find your target heart rate on the chart and practice taking it.
7. ___ Include the warm-up, aerobic, and cool-down phases during your activity.
8. ___ Begin your activity program gradually and easily.
9. ___ Remember no pain, more gain.
10. ___ Think attrACTIVE, be attrACTIVE, feel attr-ACTIVE.

Recommended Reading

Everybody's Fitness Book, Gordon W. Stewart. 3S Publishers, Santa Barbara, CA, 1982.

The Complete Sports Medicine Book for Women, Mona Shangold and Gabe Mirkin. Fireside Books, Simon and Schuster, Inc., New York, NY, 1985.

Swim for the Health of It, Ernest W. Maglischo and Cathy Ferguson Brennan. Mayfield Publishing Company, Palo Alto, CA and London, 1985.

3

Getting Started: Goal Setting

*Once we learn to accept the reality that we can't
please everyone all of the time, we can learn to
please ourselves. The rest will follow.*

Carol Cassell

In the last chapter we listed some possible goals for an
attrACTIVE WOMAN program. Some were psycho/social,
others primarily physical with psychological components. Just
listing goals does not mean that they happen in our lives—or
that all of them can happen in my particular life. When we set
a goal, we are specifying what we want to happen. There is an
art to achieving goals. Successful goals have the following characteristics:

- DESIRABLE The goal must be something you truly want
  to do, not something you feel you should do or someone
  else (partner, media, best friend, mother, kids) feels you
  should do. Consider the difference in these two statements:
  "I should walk 20 minutes every other day" and "I want to
  walk 20 minutes every other day."

- SPECIFIC The goal must clearly state what you want in
  specific rather than general terms. For example, "I want to
  be more active" is not stated in specific terms. To say "I will
  walk 20 minutes four days this week" is stated in specific
  terms and is measurable.

- FLEXIBLE The goal must allow you to be human, that is,
  not perfect. One small slip is not cause for giving up. If

your first goal isn't achieved, reevaluate the situation, perhaps return to the original goal or restate it. Do not concentrate on blaming or fault-finding. This takes a whole lot of energy which could be used to implement your goal. Beware also of what we call the "Cookie Syndrome": "I ate two cookies which was not within my goal, so I've blown it . . . I might as well just eat the whole plate full." Applied to exercise, it goes like this: "I didn't go out yesterday (or this week) so I've blown the whole program. I am a couch potato after all." No, you are just human and CAN begin again or continue with your goal because it is something you really want.

When we talk to women about what their goals for exercise might be, inevitably someone in the group says, "I will walk every morning this week." And she does—for three days. Then, due to circumstances beyond her control, she is unable to walk on the fourth morning. Her interpretation is that she is a failure, yet she accomplished so much more than the weeks before her decision to "walk every morning this week"! A more flexible goal for her would have been: "I'll walk three or four times this week" which would have allowed for different times of day and some skipped days. In this scenario, she chooses daily and she doesn't set herself up for failure while overlooking her progress and growth.

- REALISTIC Being realistic means that you start *where you are*. Appendix A lists several entry-level programs with weekly progressions. It is important to *finish one week's level before moving on to another level*. You may take four weeks to reach the level suggested for week two or three. That is fine. That is you. Build slowly and thoroughly and you won't fail, and you won't hurt.

The goal must be big enough to be challenging, but not so big it can't be accomplished. After you determine your goal, think of small steps that will get you there. Small steps taken toward a big goal will give you a feeling of satisfaction that makes the next step easier. For example, it is unrealistic to have a goal of riding a half century bicycle tour (50 miles) without breaking down this goal into daily—weekly—segments. Building s-l-o-w-l-y is the only way to such a big goal. It can be realistic or unrealistic, depending on how you break down the goal into components. The same is true of running, walking, swimming. It is not the number of miles which makes the goal realistic or not, but your approach to it. You are in charge. Focusing on the short-term goals is satisfying, realistic, and lots of fun.

One of the most successful aspects of having an attrACTIVE WOMAN group is the sharing time it allows. During the goal-setting session the group is particularly helpful in determining what is realistic and how to be flexible about goals. Here a woman discovers what goals work for her in a nurturing and supporting environment.

ESTABLISHING PERSONAL GOALS

Goals can be physical, emotional, spiritual, or perhaps combinations of all three. If the following examples fit your needs, decide how often you are able to meet the goal (three times a week, once a day?). Deciding this is important because it makes your goal measurable and keeping track of your progress and/or stumbling blocks gives you information you need for yourself.

I will walk for 30 minutes . . .
I will relax for 10 minutes . . .
I will change a negative thought about myself into a positive one . . .
I will do stretching exercises before my aerobic activity . . .
I will include vegetables in my daily food choices . . .

Now that you have had an opportunity to consider your own personal goal or goals, it is time to make a commitment to yourself *in writing*. The word, or idea of "commitment" is frightening to some women, so here is a simple format to follow. Fill out the EIGHT WEEK GOAL sheet and one WEEKLY GOAL sheet to be used each week as you move along.

EIGHT WEEK GOAL

I am a unique and special person and I will commit to caring for myself. I'll commit to an aerobic level of activity for the next eight weeks. In that time I will be aerobically active by _____ (name aerobic activity, i.e., walking, cycling, square dancing) for _____ (time) and will do this (these) activity _____ times per week.

As recognition of having achieved this, I will _____ (name a "reward" for myself).

This is my special way of celebrating my body and caring for myself.

_____ (signature)
_____ (date)

WEEKLY GOAL

Because I care about my whole self, I will commit myself to the following this week:
1. I will be aerobically active _____ times.
2. The activity (activities) I have picked is _____ .
3. I will keep track of the time I am active and my feelings before and after my activity. I will describe their kind and intensity. I will note important thoughts I had while _____ (name the activity).

This is my special way of renewing myself.

_____ (signature)
_____ (date)

Note: Other sheets for additional weeks of the program with diverse commitments are in appendix E.

In order to keep track of your goal we strongly urge keeping a training log. Yes, training log. Not exercise log. Words make a difference in how you perceive what you are doing; for years "exercise" has come to mean "drudgery" and all those "shoulds" that aren't very helpful. "Training" has a good, strong, serious tone which describes well what you're doing for yourself.

Every month or two you might decide to focus on a different goal within your general goal of sustained aerobic activity. For example, attention to better coordination and form, or flexibility through stretching. Perhaps you want to go farther or faster. These sub-goals can all be addressed as you progress in your program.

BARRIERS TO OUR GOALS

Since we have completed discussion on the reasons to get involved with a regular aerobic program, let's discuss all of the "Inhibitors to Exercise" (commonly known to us as excuses!!). This is where reality sets in . . .

- I'm too fat.
- It's too cold.
- It's too hot.
- I don't want to mess up my hair.
- I can't afford to belong to a spa.
- I'm too uncoordinated.
- It's too rainy.
- It's too dry.
- I don't want anyone to see me.
- I don't "do sweat."
- I don't have the right clothes.
- I'm too slow.
- I'm scared of dogs.
- I'm too lazy.
- It's too muggy, smoggy, foggy.
- It's too high.
- I have allergies.
- etc., etc., etc.!

Yes, these all are excuses. We used to make attempts at problem solving for each of them but now we realize that the list is infinite, and while a person is in an excuse mode there is no way of rationalizing with them. It is like banging our heads against the wall with no success. We would come up with a solution to a problem and would be hit head on with a "Yes, but, . . ." If you are stuck here with an endless list of excuses, simply put the book down, don't be hard on yourself and try again another time.

Physical Barriers

If you happen to be a woman who is differently abled, the chances are that you can get involved in aerobic and anaerobic activities too. Contact the National Handicapped Sports and Recreation Association, Suite 201, 1200 Fifteenth Street NW,

Washington, D.C. 20005, for specific information about programs and activities in your area which meet your particular interests and your situation. For outdoor interests like kayaking and rock climbing contact the Cooperative Wilderness Handicapped Outdoor Group (C.W.HOGs), Box 8118, Idaho State University, Pocatello, Idaho 83209.

There is exciting new news for women who struggle with diabetes mellitus. Aerobic activity is an essential part of your total well-being—both mentally and physically. Your physician and registered dietitian can outline the appropriate balance of activity, food, and insulin to meet your individual needs and interests. For more information contact the Diabetes Center, Inc., P.O. Box 739, Wayzata, MN 55391. (For further specific information try *Diabetes and Exercise*, by Marion J. Franz, M.S., R.D., from the same address as the Diabetes Center).

Time Barriers

The number one reason women give for not being active is "no time." In this day and age, time is an invaluable resource and so we will choose to address the problem of "no time" in more depth.

We have been in a quandary concerning this problem for several years. There are numerous short-term solutions, like use your lunch hour time, take a run instead of a walk (it takes less time), put a stationary bike near the phone and make your calls while you cycle, or join the health club which is in your neighborhood so it takes less time getting there—the list goes on and on. It has become apparent these solutions are simply a band-aid for a much deeper and more troubling problem.

There are only 24 hours in a day, not one minute more or less. It seems a little funny when someone says "I'll just make the time"—it takes a pretty special person (God) to be able to "make time." Truly it isn't "time" that is the issue. It has become clear to us that the real issue is priorities. These same women who have "no time" to be active are career people who run a company and a household, taxi kids from school to dental appointments, to music lessons, and on to soccer practice, while leading the Chamber of Commerce and preparing three square meals a day at home. They are the givers and caretakers of the world who have time, or take the time, for anyone and everyone but themselves. If you see yourself in this scenario, please step back a moment and take a look. Taking care of yourself will ultimately make you healthier and stronger for all the roles you play in life—career person, mother, spouse, Girl Scout Leader, homemaker, council woman, etc. It can be an investment in yourself which grows and matures with taking time. Consider taking time for you as self-interest and self-respect, rather than thinking of yourself as being selfish. We think not being able to take time for oneself is a very "female" problem. This is because centuries and many cultures have assigned the role of nurturing to women—exclusively. If you took care of others, then you were feminine. One's identity was tied up in a role. Today, nurturing is an activity appropriate for and expected of both men and women. It is a function of human beings, rather than an identity for one sex. This concept frees women to explore their own self-worth and interests and develop self-esteem which is not dependent on a role. In fact it is the very core of a healthy woman. When you believe enough in yourself you will take the time to take care of yourself.

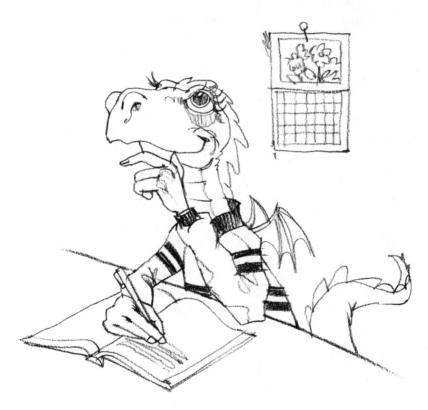

If you haven't given yourself time before, it will feel awkward at first. But the more you take some activity time for yourself, the more comfortable it will become. Begin with one day at a time. It might help to simply say to yourself "I'm going to take time for myself to be aerobically active today." See what happens; allow yourself the experience and sense how it feels— you might be as pleasantly surprised as we were! The Chinese said it this way, "A journey of a thousand miles begins with a single step."

All of this sounds so smooth. But life is not always so smooth. Weekly we hear women in the program say, "I didn't have time. I had to _____." Or "I was so tired after work that I just went to bed." Etc. Etc. There will be barriers to your goals. Look at them. What are they? What can you do about them?

BARRIERS TO BEING ACTIVE
People as Barriers

Even loving and understanding people can fall into the barrier category. If they do, ignoring them as real barriers won't help. Assessing the "who" and "why" is an important first step in getting on with solving the problem. In most cases the person is not intentionally trying to be malicious or become a barrier.

MARVEL I remember while in graduate school I was doing a lot of running. I decided to train for a marathon—my mileage was high; I had a flexible schedule; and I had met this wonderful, energetic, and fun-loving man (who was handsome to boot!) to run with. What a terrific set up! Well, almost. All summer long we trained diligently, building our mileage while sharing great companionship in the mountains of northern Utah. Into the fall we were running 50 to 60 mile weeks—I'll never forget my first 20 mile run. What a sense of power! I was one lean, mean, running machine! Two weeks before the race he wasn't feeling well . . . one week before it was clear he would not be able to run the marathon. How terrible—we had trained so hard all summer. When he finally told me he would be unable to go he added "Please Marvel, don't go without me. Wait until we can run our first marathon together." I'll never forget his hurt look. I was so disappointed and my insides were burning, but outwardly I smiled, and ever so compassionately said "Of course I wouldn't consider it without you. We'll do one next spring." He sighed, smiled, and said "I just knew you would understand, Marvel." I quickly stuffed all the feelings of disappointment and frustration way, way, down. It wasn't until months later (and my handsome running partner was history!) that I figured out what had happened. He had wanted me to wait, but I was the one who shoved my needs and wants away and put someone else's needs before mine. It wasn't so much that I was manipulated, but I allowed myself to be manipulated. It was my responsibility to take care of myself—I make the decisions. Several years later I decided to train for another marathon—this time alone! Again, building my mileage diligently over the summer, feeling strong when another man swept me off my running feet! This time with a proposal for marriage . . . alas, the morning of the marathon I was on top of Pajarito Mountain being married. So, I've been running for 18 years and still no marathon. Oh well, live and learn. Maybe the third time's a charm! Well, in time for the second printing of attrACTIVE WOMAN, I did it! I celebrated my second wedding anniversary by running a marathon. My husband supported me through my training and ran with me occasionally and cheered me on through the finish line. I feel good about it!

• • •

Often family people can become barriers, so we can ask ourself: Who gets in the way of my plan? How do I let them take charge of my plans? How can I talk to them about this problem? Am I willing to problem solve around this topic of my need to get active? Are there family members who might want to join me swimming, walking, etc.? Are there family members able to prepare meals? Or wait until a mealtime convenient for me? A change in my plans does affect others; give them time to adjust. Problem solve *with* them (instead of "laying down the new law"). No need to stop my program after the first grumble (or fifth!). Recognizing that this is difficult can pave the way for a gradual acceptance of the new and changing you.

Sometimes it is our friends who find our changing lifestyle difficult to accept. Which friends are barriers? Are they at my work place? Church/synagogue? Friends of my spouse or partner? *How* do they act as barriers? Do they assume that if I change I expect them to change too? What could my response be to them? (Practice different responses. Write them down—

then come up with some good ones to try "live".) Why do I think they act this way? Do I really want to give them the power to stop me from my goals?

Places as Barriers

Having an activity which is convenient to home or office increases the success of your commitment. Knowing you are as safe as possible is an important consideration in choosing "what" and "where." Can I do my activity IN my home? Can I do it in my home sometimes? Is the facility where I train convenient to my house? Is there a place to shower? Take care of my hair? Is my training area safe? Can I make it safer? Can I go with someone? Do I get too cold or hot here? What other clothing could help with this problem? Do I know where telephones are in my training area? Do I carry change with me for emergency phone calls; do I carry I.D.? Can I enhance the atmosphere with my own music or tapes?

Things as Barriers

Not having proper equipment can be a huge barrier to a successful program. Jogging/running/walking: Number one priority—good shoes and socks. Layered clothing. Head and hand covering in cold weather. Rain gear. Sunscreen. Sweat band (perspiration in the eyes stings!). Swimming: goggles and proper suit (nylon or lycra which is high cut—no deep cleavage to catch water and hold you back), swimmers' shampoo and conditioner (to deal with chlorine damage problems), possibly ear/nose plugs, cap (if your hair is shoulder length). Some prefer to do laps with a snorkel. That's fine; it's not cheating—it's being able to breathe comfortably. Outdoors: sun block. Cycling: Number one priority—a good helmet. Gloves, touring shorts or those "ugly black shorts" (they are more comfortable and save your bottom—which is precious and worth saving). Glasses (for sun blocking and assorted "stuff" getting in your eyes). Water bottles (2), frame pump, spare tube, patch kit. Sweat band. Sunscreen. Layered clothing (don't ride very bare skinned, if you fall you will regret it). See appendix B for more details and for recommended equipment for other sports.

Weather Barriers

Certainly at times weather—wind, rain, snow, sleet, cold, heat—can be a barrier to the aerobic activities we might have

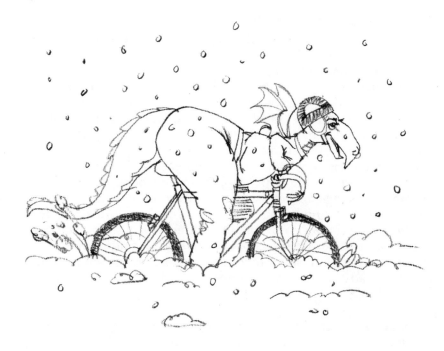

chosen. Certainly having the proper equipment and clothing is a big help. Planning for foul weather days by having alternate activities such as indoor swimming, a stationary cycle, or treadmill will work. Something we have learned is that if you continue your activity throughout the year your body can adjust to the climate. Your body adjusts slowly with the changing seasons, particularly with the drop and rise in temperature. If we allow ourselves to gain wisdom from our bodies when they are faced with inclement weather there is much to be learned.

MARVEL One of the greatest wisdoms I gained was while canoeing on an extensive trip which included 14 days and nights of non-stop rain. I learned I've never been so wet that I couldn't get dry! Facing barriers can be a humbling experience of facing how little control we have over nature and how we have to flow with it—not fight it.

• • •

The Final Barrier: Ourselves

Often we overlook one of the greatest barriers of all, when learning new activities—ourselves. No, not our physical capabilities: Can I actually DO this sport? CAN I play this way? Nor is it a question of our intellectual ability to grasp the concepts or understand how an activity is performed. It is our expectations of ourselves. Somewhere along the line many of us picked up the message that we have to do things perfectly or not at all. It is the old "all or nothing" thinking . . . it has to be 100 percent right or not at all. Women often don't cut themselves enough slack for being human and being human does not mean being perfect. Anyone out there know anyone who gets paid for being human (i.e., a professional human being)? Or are we all a bunch of amateur human beings just learning how? We can be so critical of ourselves; certainly we wouldn't treat others in the same manner! This all-or-nothing, perfectionist's attitude is sometimes referred to as black or white thinking.

MARVEL In a group meeting once, a woman struggling with an issue described her options as "feeling like it was black or white—I lose no matter what." Another woman asked her if there wasn't any grey in between? She replied that grey didn't feel good and the rest of the women agreed it felt dreary, down, and hopeless. After group I was out running and contemplating about black and white thinking when I struck onto something— if black is on one end and white symbolizes the other end, then where are all the colors in between? What about yellow, fuchsia, blue, green, turquoise, brown, red, burgundy, rose? As I ran, it seemed to me, there are subtle colors of infinite options of our feelings between the extremes of black and white. Sense what green feels like? violet? electric blue? Thinking in black and white about what a rainbow is is a sure road to failure. Thinking colors bursts open an array of feelings in depths, intensities, variability, and hues we may never have known existed. I ran on. It became clear that when a woman recognizes options, life doesn't automatically become blissful. I could hardly wait until group the next week!

• • •

Perfectionism is a setup for failure. We can guarantee it if we expect to be perfect. Go easy on yourself.

Of special note concerning barriers—pain can be a barrier. We've mentioned it before—we'll mention it again: we don't believe in "no pain, no gain." We believe in "no pain, more gain." Pain is different from discomfort which can generally be dealt with. Pain is a barrier which is a signal. Pay attention. Be gentle and loving with yourself. You're worth it.

SOLVING OUR PROBLEMS, REWARDING OURSELVES

After barriers are identified, then problem solving is in order. Are these long-range barriers, or short-range ones? The simplest, believe it or not, are monetary ones. Some equipment can be purchased second hand, through catalogs (though not always cheapest) or saved for. But people problems take a bit of finesse, thought, and time. People problems are not insurmountable problems—there are "different strokes for different folks," and different techniques for different ones. Most frequently we find that women allow people to sabotage their fitness program. **You can still be a warm caring person who thinks of others and maintains an aerobic program for yourself.**

If other people are your top priority in life, then look at it this way: if you are energized and more "together," you'll have more to offer them.

Not all barriers can be eliminated. Some can be gotten around, jumped over, climbed slowly . . . dismantled.

What technique will I use? Again, BE SPECIFIC. Barriers have a way of reappearing. What will I do *now?* Your brain will be a big help to you in this problem solving. Talking to your active friends may give you ideas. Read. A firm commitment to solving the problem—dealing with the barrier—is the vital beginning point.

Finally, it is important that you review your progress with your goals. Keep track. Write it down. Don't expect that you will remember what you did when, how far you went, or how fast. When you write it down you are being gentle with your memory. Give yourself a break.

Speaking of which, how about some rewards for yourself?

- a long hot bath (with scent)
- time to read a novel (or a chapter)
- a movie with someone special
- listening to a lovely song
- reading poetry
- buying flowers for yourself
- looking at a picture book
- going to a museum
- having breakfast alone . . . or with a friend (lifestyle determines which would be the greater "treat")
- a long-distance phone call
- a massage
- a nature hike
- an article of sport clothing
- browse in a bookstore, antique shop, fabric store

Rewards can be inexpensive or very dear; take a few minutes or hours. Whichever they are, they say to yourself "Good job!" You'd say that to your friends or family if they were moving toward their goals, why not be as supportive and loving toward yourself?

Finally, a note on a calendar may suffice to keep track of frequency, but we'd recommend writing down how you *felt* about your training; what insights you had, what surprises occurred. These are as important as data about time, distance, intensity, frequency. They tell you about yourself as a whole woman (more about emotions later) . . . someone becoming daily more and more attrACTIVE.

Recommended Reading

Running for Health and Beauty: A Complete Guide for Women; Kathryn Lance. Bobbs-Merrill Company, Inc., Indianapolis, New York, 1978.

4

Food Glorious Food!

When it comes to weight, people can't accept a happy ending that leaves us different shapes and sizes. To me, a happy ending is when someone can accept her body as it is.

Susan Wooley

Do you ever feel like there is absolutely nothing left to eat that isn't carcinogenic, going to plug your arteries with fat, create endless yeast infections, cause chemical brain imbalances, or infest your intestines with heebie-jeebies?! Is there anything safe that a sane woman might find palatable? Has all the fun been blown out of eating for you? Take heart—we plan to blow the frustration out of making food choices so some joy is returned to eating.

There are endless reasons why we eat—nearly all social situations involve partaking of food and libations: religious festivities, cultural ceremonies and events, holidays, weddings, parties, etc. Occasionally we even eat when we are hungry! We are hard pressed to think of events that do not include eating. Food is a consistent part of our daily living. The food marketing industry claims that people make an average of 30 decisions per day concerning food. For many, food is the answer to emotional cries for help—when we are lonely, frustrated, angry, and hurt, or when we are on emotional highs—feeling exuberant and happy. Many of us learned at a very young age that food is a reward when things are not going well. Do you ever remember receiving a lollipop after getting a shot at the doctor's office or a sweet when you scraped your knee? Few of the reasons we eat have anything to do with fueling our bodies with energy to keep the "motor" running or to be physically active.

Unfortunately many women feel much pressure about food and what they "should" or "shouldn't" be eating. It seems much of the "Joy of Eating" has been lost—overruled by feelings of guilt about eating, and self-disapproval concerning our body size and shape and what we "should" or "shouldn't" look like. (This is another opportunity to evaluate when we are "should-on" by ourselves or others.) There are endless rules about what we can't ever have because it is bad for us or it is "junk" food. It seems impossible to eat without the feeling of guilt cropping up and taking all the fun out of what can be a very enjoyable experience.

In this chapter we plan to simplify the information about choices of eating. As a result you might begin feeling less guilty and bring to yourself some of the enjoyment of a healthy, nurturing process.

Nutrition is a fascinating science in this day and age. Scientists are daily grasping new knowledge concerning the biochemistry of how our bodies utilize food and how our daily choices play important roles in the prevention of chronic diseases, affect our emotions and our daily living. We are in the infancy stages of what there is yet to be learned.

Regardless of the technological advancements in the science of nutrition, fallacies abound and there is endless nutrition misinformation, often based solely on the zeal to sell a product. (Note that in many states and provinces anyone can call themselves a nutritionist; to be sure, ask if their degree is from an accredited university or if they are a registered dietitian.) Hence, mountains of conflicting information are available. The unfortunate end result is that a person is left with the feeling of overwhelming confusion and frustration.

Of the 10 leading causes of death in Canada and the United States, seven are nutrition related including heart disease, diabetes, and cancer. There is no doubt that these are serious public health problems, but what we view as the number one nutrition problem for women in these countries is dieting—not overweight, or obesity, nor even "overfat"—but dieting!

DIETING AND DISORDERED EATING

Dieting is a chronic and often lifetime problem for women. It is one of the most self-destructive activities we know. Dieting is the epitome of a lack of self-acceptance and low self-esteem. Studies by the National Institute of Health indicate that about

50 percent of women are on a diet at least two times per year. At any one time in the U.S. it is conservatively estimated that 28 percent of people are on diets and closer to half of people are "restrictive" eaters. Laurel Mellin of the University of California, San Francisco, found that 31 percent of nine-year-old girls and 81 percent of ten-year-old girls have already been on a calorie-restrictive diet. There is an overwhelming "fear of fat" for girls and women and it is making us emotionally and mentally sick. The incidences of eating disorders—anorexia nervosa, bulimia nervosa, compulsive eating, and bingeing—are estimated to affect anywhere from 15 percent to 25 percent of college-age women. Besides women suffering diagnosed eating disorders, there are millions of women of all ages, races, religions, shapes, and sizes waging war on themselves.

The war is: a relentless attempt to reshape their bodies to the impossible societal expectations of "beauty." (Mind you, this is a very fickle definition of "beauty." Remember Rembrant? Rubens? Rodin? If we followed their concept of beauty, millions would start eating today!)

The battle armament includes: wired jaws, stapled stomachs, cutout chunks of intestines, suctioning fat from specific areas (ouch), plastic sweat wraps, vomiting (ipecac used when desperate!), laxatives, billions of diet pills (in 1983 there were one billion tablets of phenylpropanolamine sold over the counter specifically as appetite suppressants—at a cost of more than 150 million dollars and that is just one drug!), and above all, endless diets (98 percent of which don't work).

The outcome is: — failure, after failure, after failure!
— battle scars of abused bodies
— strangled self-images
— battered bodies, spirits, and emotions.

Diets (and dieting techniques) simply don't work. If they did, wouldn't everybody use one and be *slim-sexy-beautiful?* *(that* glossy, marketed—very limited—image of women makes *us* feel sick.)

The Yo-Yo Syndrome
The diet industry in the U.S. is a multi-billion dollar business—it is the only business we know of that survives on its own failures! Have you even gotten what was promised? If it

sounds too good to be true, it probably is. Women get on the dieting roller coaster and the ride doesn't stop. They are caught in the yo-yo syndrome of gain-lose-gain-lose-gain. We fondly think of this as the "rhythm method of girth control"! Dieting is the "curse of the eating class." It affects nearly everyone, not just those dieting—have you ever lived with a dieter?!

Let us explain—it goes something like this: A woman is told directly or indirectly by someone or "something" she read or saw, that she needs to lose weight; she is too fat and is unacceptable the way she is. When a person thinks this way it may be self-imposed or come from outside put-downs—in any case it is self-believed. Obviously a person begins feeling insecure and inadequate; then comes the dangerous next step. Anything that is not going right in her life is blamed on being too fat and/or ugly. So she begins a diet to solve her problems. It might be a diet from a magazine, a book off the best-seller list, her physician, a T.V. advertisement, or a self-imposed restrictive eating regime. Whatever the source, the diet begins and the first thing she loses is her sense of humor! Dieting is so depriving and has so many rules of what you can and can't have that it is as if a person is on a diet because they have been "bad" and this deprivation is a form of punishment. Generally a person begins to lose weight—alas! The magic is happening—but what is it that she is losing? A combination of water, muscle tissue, and fat tissue. The scale *only* measures weight, it does not measure what is being lost. *The scale is not a tool which can measure whether we are healthy, fit, or the right size—or beautiful!* Physically, it gives us the information of total body weight *only*. Emotionally, we allow it to give us all sorts of messages like "I am a good or a bad person today because I have lost or gained weight." It seems to us that women give far too much power in determining self-worth to a scale. Think for a moment. What messages of worth or accomplishment do you let the scale give you?

If you are caught in the "Dreaded Scale Syndrome" we urge you to choose as one of your first goals abandoning the scale—literally and figuratively. Trust yourself to measure your weight and your value. Concentrate on being and looking attractive without it. Try it for a week, or two, or a month.

Anyway, back to the dieting saga. You begin to lose weight and your body (being pretty sharp and wise) begins to react—in many ways. When you are not eating enough food it "slows down" internally and becomes very efficient with the fuel (food) it has to use. This is known as a lowered metabolic rate. So your body becomes adjusted to not getting enough to eat yet surviving very efficiently. As you lose muscle tissue your body does not need as much energy (calories) because muscle tissue requires much more energy than fat tissue does to function.

Since restrictive eating is so far from reality, you eventually eat something that is on the "forbidden list" and guilt sets in (not instant globs of fat, as imagined). Sometimes it triggers an eating binge because "I messed up anyway so I might as well go all the way." Or you get to the "right weight" and go off the diet or something interrupts the dieting activity. When you go back to your regular eating habits it is inevitable you will gain weight back—this time what is the weight made up of? The water you lost will have returned and the weight you regain will most likely be fat tissue.

So the cycle of dieting begins and the failures start adding up. You are now fatter than you were before. Maybe you don't weigh more, since fat weighs less than muscle—but you take up more space and chances are physically and emotionally you don't feel very well. The more often you yo-yo diet, the LOWER your metabolic rate, the easier the weight gain is, and the less and less you have to eat to still gain weight. Not a very good bargain for the price of quick weight loss diets and fads.

It is a cruel cartoon that overweight people overeat—more likely they overDIET! A person with a higher percent of lean body tissue often eats much more than someone overweight. Haven't you sat down to eat with lean active women and been amazed at how much fuel they can consume? (and felt more than a little jealous?)

MARVEL On numerous occasions I have had comments directed at me of "Oh, you're one of those!—eat whatever you want and never have a problem in the world . . . " and it is usually expressed with an overtone of hostility. We'll bet that these active women who eat what they want (and enjoy it) have not recently been roller coaster dieting. They have problems— as all women do—but they are likely not to link them with body weight. Self-image, self-worth, is placed elsewhere.

•　•　•

Dieting is a vicious, mean cycle and it simply does not work. And the price is very high indeed. Your self-worth gets all wound up in your (or someone else's) body image and your experience of failure at dieting. From this perspective it is no wonder that people will try anything to lose weight. Very reminiscent of Cinderella's sisters doing anything to get into that glass slipper! The reality is not "fitting in," but an overwhelming sense of helplessness and hopelessness.

Another popular fallacy is that an overweight person is mentally unstable and needs to eat to solve their problems. Often a person is trying to feed an emotional hunger rather than a physical one, but there is no correlation between obesity and mental illness. Nearly everyone eats for emotional reasons at one time or another and there is nothing really wrong with it on occasion. Some women have been compulsively over or undereating to mask all their feelings, and if you see yourself in this place, seek professional help.

Somewhere, somehow, we have to begin eliminating diets rather than food. If you can harness all the energy and work that goes into dieting and put it into nurturing yourself, you will be on the right track. We have to quit worrying about being fat and start being fit! The key is to give yourself permission to eat so your body is nurtured, your metabolic rate isn't lowered, and you have the strength to be physically active—then it is possible to develop lean body tissue.

Maybe you identify with the yo-yo syndrome and suspect you have gained more fat than muscle tissue and your metabolic rate has been lowered by all the dieting. It is not a hopeless situation—there is a way out of this vicious cycle. You will need to:

- give up dieting as a way of life
- be aerobically active as outlined in chapter 2
- become consistent in the amount of food you eat as outlined on pages 72-73
- eat on a regular basis so your body can count on being fed and won't react by lowering your metabolic rate
- retire the scale
- ask for support from others (Overeaters Anonymous for those who over- or undereat has helped thousands—see page 118.)
- be gentle with yourself
- *take one day at a time*

None of these are easy if you have been a chronic dieter. It may be frightening to try things so radically different than what you have been used to. Give yourself permission to get support and ask for help whenever you need or want to.

If you do decide to follow or join a weight management program (not a diet!) use the checklist below. This way you can be sure it is a sound and healthy way of treating your body.

WEIGHT MANAGEMENT PROGRAM CHECKLIST

If you think it is necessary to enroll in a weight management program, use this checklist. This is a list for women who are not *emotion-focused* eaters. When selecting a program be sure it includes all of the following components:

_____ targets fat loss—not just pounds lost

_____ if it includes weight loss, it aims for a very gradual weight change of 1/2 to 1 1/2 pounds per week

_____ IS BASED ON REGULAR AEROBIC ACTIVITY

_____ includes the minimum amount of a variety of foods from all four food groups

_____ contains at least 10 calories for every 1 pound body weight per day (i.e., a 140 pound woman needs 1,400 calories per day)—preferably it does not have you count calories but has you choose foods from *all* the food groups (see pages 72-73).

_____ encourages plenty of liquids

_____ has a strong component of building self-esteem and changing eating habits

_____ avoids large amounts of vitamin, mineral, and dietary supplements

_____ utilizes relaxation and stress management techniques

_____ is led by qualified personnel (i.e., registered dietitian)

Without healthy eating habits, all the aerobic activity, stress management techniques, and physical exams you could take will do little good in your pursuit of wellness. Wise food choices are the basis for physical health and total well-being and your delicate physical balance begins with food. Remember food is fuel, *food is not the enemy.*

The key concepts to keep in mind concerning food are variety and moderation. These are the basis of good nutrition and a balanced eating plan as it is outlined in the Healthy Eating Guide on pages 72-73.

Enjoy Your Fun Foods

There is nothing you have to totally eliminate from your food choices. We intentionally do not refer to "junk" or "bad" foods but prefer to talk about "fun" foods or treats. As soon as a food is labelled as "bad" or "forbidden" it takes mental energy to avoid it and then when you do eat it, you have broken a rule and have become a "bad girl." How many times have you said just before eating something "Oh, I really shouldn't but . . . "? It is better to simply give yourself the freedom to have any food and then enjoy your fun food occasionally. Certainly there will be less guilt involved with eating and it would be far easier than restricting yourself and giving all that energy and power to a forbidden food. This is not an open license to eat five chocolate bars at a time, but you will be far less likely to do so if you give yourself permission to enjoy one sometimes.

Maximize Your Nutrient Intake

In order to get a healthy intake of carbohydrates, protein, fat, vitamins, and minerals, it is essential to follow the basic keys of variety and moderation. We could go into all of the details of percent of calories you need from carbohydrate, protein, and fat; the number of grams of fiber required to be healthy; the ratio of polyunsaturated to saturated fat, etc., but it gets so complicated that it is unrealistic to make it work in our busy lives. Now wouldn't you rather be out playing than calculating the percent of kilocalories from monounsaturated fat in your next meal? We have eased the decision-making of food choices by grouping foods according to their nutrient content so you won't miss any important nutrients and using a concept of nutrient density—simply, what nutrient value do you get for the number of calories consumed?

The eating guide outlined here will minimize your hassle in making food choices and maximize your nutrient intake so you too can experience the energizing benefits and enjoyment of eating. Your energy level is in your control more than you may know. ENJOY!

A special note for those trying to gain weight: we respect the fact that you also suffer from stereotypes, like, "she eats like a bird," or "she probably hates food." Some thin women, like their plump sisters, falsely connect self-worth and strength to diet issues, thereby thinking of themselves as "lightweights" and "frail" in the world. These women also feel "bad" about themselves for what they don't eat and the weight they don't gain. Many thin women may eat properly and in sufficient amounts, but they don't utilize the food in the same way as other women. Again, we want to point out it is not a certain body weight or rigid percentage of body fat that equals health, but more importantly, how one feels and how one's body functions. Do you have the strength and energy to do the things you like to do? If not, proper food choices can help you to greater physical well-being. The following guide can be your guide too. Your choices will include larger quantities of food.

For a more personalized plan than the guide which follows, see a Registered Dietitian.

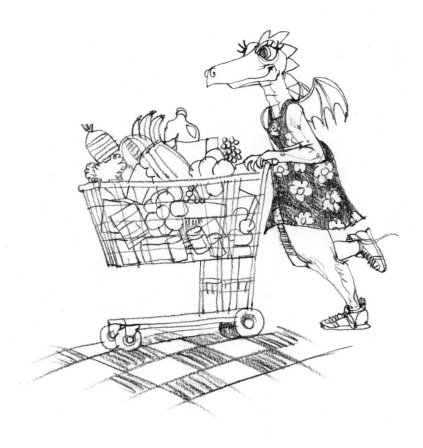

FOR HEALTHY WOMEN Minimum Daily	ANYTIME Low in fat, salt, or sugar. Vegetables, fruits and grains in this column are high in fiber.	IN MODERATION Medium amounts of fat, salt, or sugar.	NOW AND THEN High in fat, salt, or sugar.
VEGETABLE/ FRUIT **4 or more servings** 1 vitamin C rich 1 dark green leafy 2 others *1 serving = ½ cup, 1 piece, or 4 oz. juice*	All vegetables and fruits except those listed at right. Applesauce, unsweetened Chilies Fruit juices, unsweetened Potatoes, white or sweet Vegetable juices, unsalted	Avocado Guacamole Vegetables, canned with salt Vegetable juice, salted	Fruits, canned in syrup Fruit juices, sweetened
GRAIN **4 or more servings *1 serving = 1 slice bread, 1 ounce cereal, or ½ cup cooked pasta or rice*	Barley Bread, whole grain Cereals, whole grain Oatmeal Pasta, whole wheat, spinach Popcorn, plain Rice, brown Tortillas, corn Tortillas, whole wheat	Biscuits Bread, white Cereals, granola Cereals, refined Corn bread Crackers, whole wheat or soda, unsalted Muffins Pancakes Pasta Popcorn, small amount of fat and salt Rice, white Tortillas, white flour Waffles	Pretzels
MILK PRODUCTS **3 servings** *1 serving = 1 cup milk, 1 cup yogurt, or 1½ ounces cheese*	Buttermilk Cheese, farmer or pot Cottage cheese, low-fat Milk, low-fat (1%) non-fat dry skim	Cheese, low-fat or part skim Cocoa, made with skim milk Cottage cheese, regular Ice milk Milk, low-fat (2%) Yogurt, low-fat, frozen Yogurt, low-fat, plain	Cheese, hard or processed Eggnog Ice cream Milk, whole Yogurt, fruit flavored

72

GUIDE TO HEALTHY EATING

FOR HEALTHY WOMEN Minimum Daily	ANYTIME Low in fat, salt, or sugar. Vegetables, fruits and grains in this column are high in fiber.	IN MODERATION Medium amounts of fat, salt, or sugar.	NOW AND THEN High in fat, salt, or sugar.
MEAT/ ALTERNATES **2 servings** 1 meat, fish or poultry 1 vegetable protein *1 serving = 2 ounces meat, fish, poultry or 1 cup cooked beans or ¼ cup nuts*	Vegetable: dried beans, peas, lentils Fish: cod, flounder, haddock, perch, sole, water-packed tuna Poultry: chicken or turkey *(no skin)* Meat: cuts or ground meat labelled very lean	Eggs Fish: herring, mackerel, salmon, sardines, oil-packed tuna, shellfish Meat: flank, leg, loin, round, rump, tenderloin, most veal Vegetable: nuts *(including pinon)* refried beans, soy beans, peanut butter	Fish and poultry: deep fried Meat: brisket, chuck, chorizo, cold cuts, corned beef, frankfurters, ground beef or pork, hamburger, jerky, liver, rib roasts, rib steaks, sausage, spare ribs, untrimmed meats
COMBINATION FOODS	Mixtures of "Anytime" foods. Salad: mixed fruit, tossed greens Soup: vegetable	Beef and vegetable stew Burrito Chile con carne with beans Chile, green or red Enchiladas Lasagna Pizza Posole Salad, three bean Spaghetti *Prepare these items with lean meats, low-fat cheese, and minimal fat and salt.*	Chicken a la king Chile relleno Fast food: hamburgers, sandwiches, main dishes Macaroni and cheese Meat loaf Pot pies Soup, canned and dried Stroganoff Tacos Tamales Tostadas
OTHERS *Provide few nutrients. Many are high in calories.* *Eat as needed for more energy and enjoyment.*	Alcoholic beverages, bacon, butter, cake, candy, chocolate*, coffee*, cookies, cream, cream cheese, french fries, gravies, jams, jellies, lard, margarine, mayonnaise, olives, pickles, pies, potato chips, presweetened cereals, sauerkraut, salad oils, soda pop*, sopaipillas, ice cream, stuffing, sugar, syrups, tea*, tortilla chips *May be high in caffeine. **Active women need to add more grains—6 to 12 servings daily.		

Food or Drink	Amount	Vegetable/ Fruit
Total Number of Servings Eaten		
Minimum Servings Needed		4+
Difference		

*6-12 servings for active women

DIRECTIONS:

1. In the left hand column list everything you ate and drank for the last 24 hours. Include the amount. Remember the extras . . . salad dressing, butter, sour cream, etc.
2. Using the Guide to Healthy Eating above, find what food group each item you ate is in. Find the corresponding serving size. For example: 1½ cups yogurt = 1½ servings milk, 1 cup broccoli = 2 servings vegetables, 1½ cups cooked pasta = 3 servings grain.

EVALUATION GUIDE

Grain	Milk Products	Meat/ Alternates	Water/ Clear Liquids
4+*	3	2	8-10**

** Plus 2 for every hour active

3. Find the food group column across the page and fill in the number of servings eaten.
4. Total each column.
5. Find the difference between the minimum you needed and what you actually ate.

Now you will be able to see for yourself which food groups you are lacking or overindulging in and can make choices accordingly. Note whether you are eating more choices from the 'Now and Then' category or the 'Anytime' category.

NUTRITION NOTES

The following notes will complement the food guide above and detail some nutrition and food specifics you will want to know as an attrACTIVE woman. We have chosen to discuss the items mentioned most by women such as yourselves who are pursuing active life-styles.

Alcohol

If you drink alcohol, do so in moderation and don't drive. Wine, beer, and liquor have low nutrient density (e.g., high in calories and low in nutrient content). Women sometimes cut out food when they drink alcohol because of the calorie content—this is a poor choice since your body needs more than merely calories. It is a fallacy that wine is a good source of iron and that beer is high in the B vitamins.

Alcohol will not improve your physical performance. It decreases the strength of your heart's contraction and increases your heart's oxygen demands. Alcohol decreases the amount of blood that flows to your working muscles and therefore lessens the amount of oxygen which is vital to their aerobic activity. It forces your body to perspire more so you lose water and may become dehydrated. When alcohol is in your bloodstream your muscles burn more glycogen (energy stored in muscles) and less fat, so you run out of energy sooner and cannot go as long nor as hard.

MARVEL The only time alcohol helped me in a running race was at the Toney Grove Challenge—a fourteen-mile race. Seven grueling miles up to a mountain lake, and seven miles down. Few women entered this "fun" run, those who did were strong. There was one woman from out of state who said she was in her best condition ever and thought she had a good chance of having a Personal Record Time and of placing in the winning category. I knew she was a little out of my league, but I decided to challenge myself to pace with her for as long as I could hang on. From the start I did everything to stay with her. When she sped up or slowed down I followed. When she passed someone I passed also.

At about six miles she started to pull away and I couldn't keep up. At the turn-around her husband, who was coaching her from the car gave her a can of beer. While she was drinking I passed her. I never saw her again until the awards ceremony when I was receiving the first place trophy and a certificate for holding a new course record. I don't care what people say. Alcohol helped me win that race!

• • •

Artificial Sweeteners

Fructose, sorbitol, mannitol, and xylitol have all been used as substitutes for sugar in foods for people with diabetes, and all of these sweeteners provide as many or more calories as sucrose (table sugar). Some people have reported problems with diarrhea when using these products. Saccharin is a non-caloric sweetener used to sweeten beverages and foods. There has been some concern from animal studies about a correlation with cancer which has resulted in a ban of its use in some countries. Most people complain about its aftertaste. Aspartame, a synthetic combination of two protein components, is available for use as a sweetener in breakfast cereals, powdered beverages, gelatins, puddings, fillings, whipped toppings, and chewing gum. It has the trade name "Equal" as a tablet or powder and is very sweet and low in calories. Some people report experiencing dizziness, blurred vision, and other side effects. There is no definite conclusion that these are caused by aspartame.

We are not in the position here to argue pro or con about the safety of artificial sweeteners. Obviously not all the data is in. It would seem prudent that if you choose to use them, you do so with moderation, maybe once or twice a day, particularly for children and pregnant women. It seems the more important issue is that large scale studies have shown that such sweeteners do not prevent weight gain—a primary reason people use them. Indeed, they may stimulate appetite and promote weight gain. A study of weight gain over a six-year period of time in more than 78,000 women found those who used sugar substitutes were more likely to gain weight faster regardless of their beginning weights. Is it possible that when you use the sweeteners it leads you to overindulge in high calorie foods you might otherwise pass up? Another study found that aspartame increased feelings of hunger and decreased feelings of fullness. Once again, it appears that there is no "quick fix" to weight problems. Once again, we emphasize that calories are not the problem. A lowered metabolic rate from not consuming enough food and being underactive are the culprits.

Caffeine

Caffeine is naturally found in some plants. When food or drinks are by-products of these plants the chemical caffeine is contained in them. The most common places caffeine is found in our diet are coffee, tea, some soft drinks, and chocolate. In addition, it is found in the over-the-counter drugs like diet pills and certain pain relievers and allergy medications. Caffeine is a stimulant which can be addictive and related to increased or irregular heartbeats, headaches, trembling, nervousness, and irritability. It can increase your urine output which puts you at greater risk for dehydration. Studies have indicated moderate amounts of caffeine (four cups of coffee) can trigger panic attacks in people who are prone to them. There also is an association between caffeine ingestion and certain cancers. As caffeine consumption increases so does the need for more calcium.

Caffeine will probably not help you in competition. It causes your body to produce more adrenaline which has some effect on how your muscles use energy but if you are in a competition your body is already producing all the adrenaline you need because of the excitement. The extra adrenaline caused by the caffeine might make you shaky which won't help, but may hinder. Having the caffeine may also cause you to have to urinate more frequently which can dehydrate your body and be a general nuisance in competition. Your training and hard work are what will improve your performance!

Calcium

Calcium is a necessary mineral for building strong bones and teeth, transmission of nerve impulses, muscle contractions and relaxations, and blood clotting. Women commonly do not get enough calcium unless they pay special attention to their food choices. Without enough dietary calcium you are particularly at risk for osteoporosis (bone thinning). Other risk factors for osteoporosis include: being Caucasian or Oriental, thin or sedentary, smoking cigarettes, drinking excessive alcohol, living to an old age, and having a family history of osteoporosis. So, there are some risk factors over which we have no control and several about which we can make life-style choices.

Being active and exercising as opposed to being sedentary will help thicken and strengthen bones if you are getting enough calcium in your diet. It is recommended you get 800 to 1,000 milligrams of calcium each day. Following menopause you will require about 1,200 to 1,500 milligrams daily. In order to do this you will need to include dairy products in your food choices, since they are such calcium-rich foods. (See appendix D) If you are unable to consume any dairy products, you will need to carefully choose other high-calcium foods and possibly take a calcium supplement (pill). Estimate about how much calcium you are getting from food by using the evaluation form and charts in appendix D; read the label carefully on the supplement package for the calcium content so you don't "oversupplement" since you are likely getting some calcium in your diet. A key here is understanding "supplement," which means in addition to your food intake, not *instead* of food. If you have had kidney stones composed of calcium you should not take calcium pills and you need to ask your doctor for advice.

Some people lack an enzyme used to digest fluid milk and they get indigestion and feel bloated when they drink milk. They can usually drink milk labelled "acidophillus" (available in most grocery stores) or purchase lactose tablets from a pharmacy to add to regular milk which will usually alleviate the problem. Often these people can enjoy buttermilk, yogurt, and cheeses without discomfort.

Carbohydrates

Many women still believe that carbohydrates and starches are "fattening"! They are not; they have less than half the calories of fats. Carbohydrates, (the complex ones) like bread, cereal, pasta, rice, potatoes, beans, and vegetables are the basis of an active woman's energy stores. The more active you are, the more of these vitamin and mineral loaded foods you need. Now, if the baked potato is merely a boat to float the butter, sour cream, and bacon bits, there is a slight problem! Enjoy your bread, spaghetti, potatoes, etc., without frying and adding extra fats.

Cholesterol

Increased amounts of cholesterol in your blood is associated with heart disease. The cholesterol in your blood comes from within your body (some of us produce more than others) and from the food you eat. Since you can't control what your body is producing, we will talk about the food sources. For people with cholesterol problems, eating less foods that have cholesterol may help. Cholesterol is found in animal products only (fatty meats, egg yolks, whole milk products); plant products contain no cholesterol. There are other dietary factors that effect the amount of cholesterol in your blood. The more fat, oil, or grease of any kind you eat will probably increase it. Saturated fats—those that are solid at room temperature like animal fats, butter, lard, or hard margarine, whether from plants or animals—and coconut and palm oils can add to the problem. Try polyunsaturated oils like safflower, soy, corn, or olive, whenever necessary. Increasing the amount of fish you eat to between two and four times a week may help. Eating certain high-fiber foods like oatmeal (or oat bran), lentils, and legumes, carrots, and apples is helpful; try to choose two servings of these foods per day.

Other things effect your blood cholesterol level: smoking increases it; a high body fat content increases it; and last, but by far not the least, regular aerobic activity is essential—it decreases your body fat if this is a problem and it can increase the HDL cholesterol which carry cholesterol away from your blood vessels.

It is a good idea to know what your blood cholesterol level is . . . it is not possible to know whether it is high or low by how you feel. A simple blood test called a blood lipid profile can detect cholesterol problems. Check with your physician, local public health department or Registered Dietician.

Cravings

Lots of women struggle with craving different foods and they feel "weak" because they crave something and are not "strong" enough to overcome it. Cravings are very real—many of us have experienced them just before menses. Rather than spending a lot of energy fighting the craving, because generally that just makes it worse, give yourself permission to have the chocolate (or whatever) and enjoy it. Often cravings are due to restrictive eating (dieting). When we suppress, we obsess. Choosing poor quality food, or not having enough complete carbohydrates can also lead to cravings. It requires following the Guide to Healthy Eating already stated and not dieting. Rarely does a craving occur due to a nutrient deficiency. Sometimes a woman craves a non-food item like chalk or corn starch and this needs medical attention. If you feel very out of control with sweets and binge on large amounts frequently, please seek out professional help for compulsive eating.

Fat

A fatty diet is high in calories (with few nutrients) and increases your risk of heart disease, cancer, and other serious problems. Choose lean meats, fish, poultry, and dried beans for protein. Select low fat cheeses, yogurts, and milk. Cut down on bacon, (fondly known as "butter on a string"!) fatty sausage, butter, margarine, mayonnaise, sauces, gravies, and salad dressings. (Are you one of those people who use lettuce merely as a means of getting the Roquefort from the plate to your lips!?) Retire the frying pan . . . bake, broil, boil, or roast instead. Limit "fast foods" which are usually high in fat . . . this doesn't mean never have a french fry again—just enjoy them occasionally.

Fiber

Try nature's "broom" by including fiber in your diet. Fiber absorbs water, aids digestion, and helps prevent constipation. Increased fiber is associated with lowered risk of some cancers and certain fiber may help lower blood cholesterol levels (see cholesterol above). Choose fresh vegetables, fruits, dried beans, and whole grains and cereals.

Iron

Iron is a trace mineral which builds red blood cells and is important for its oxygen carrying capacity. Due to a woman's regular menstrual flow she may be at risk for iron deficiency anemia (iron poor blood), which means feeling tired or weak, experiencing shortness of breath or maybe a loss of appetite. Living at higher altitudes puts greater demands on the blood supply to have more iron. It is a very simple and inexpensive test to see if you have anemia; ask your physician or local health office personnel. Sometimes a woman needs to take an iron supplement. To prevent iron deficiency anemia, choose foods rich in iron (which does not mean having to eat liver!) and follow the tips found in appendix D.

Processed Foods

Select foods close to the way Mother Nature gives them to us. Many nutrients are lost during food processing and when they are cooked. So choose orange juice instead of orange drink; a baked potato instead of potato chips; whole grain breads and cereals instead of white bread and processed cereals; instead of canned vegetables, enjoy raw or lightly steamed ones.

Salt

Go easy on salt. Most people eat more salt than they need. It is a learned taste to like more salt so by slowing down on the salt shaker we can "unlearn" it too. Cutting down may help lower your blood pressure if it is high. Use more unprocessed foods as suggested above and use less salty foods (i.e., ham, pickles, processed lunch and breakfast meats). Try seasoning with fresh herbs and spices or powders (i.e., garlic or onion powders, celery seeds).

When exercising, you will lose some salt (sodium) through perspiration (or "sweat" or "glow" or whatever you do!). This is a normal response. It is not necessary to take in more salt because your body reacts immediately by not losing as much sodium in your urine. Over time, as you become fitter, your muscles will lose less sodium and other important electrolytes when you are active. Isn't your body amazing!?

Sugar

Too many sweets may promote dental decay and mean calories with little or no nutritive value. Sugar comes in lots of forms: white sugar, brown sugar, raw sugar, cane sugar, molasses, honey, corn syrup, and fructose. It is used extensively in processing foods and you might be surprised when you read labels at the number of foods which don't taste sweet, that contain sugar (check out a ketchup label). When you cook or bake, try cutting the sugar in the recipes by one fourth. Suffice it to say: enjoy your sweets, treats, and fun foods, and choose the mainstay of your foods from the eating guide outlined earlier.

Snacks

Just about everybody snacks . . . and why not? Snacks give us a lift when we need it, particularly with the kind of hectic lifestyles many of us lead. But we bet you have heard that "snacking makes you fat." On the contrary, frequent small meals—eaten throughout the day—are much less fattening than infrequent, large ones. Enjoying a snack is not the same as compulsive eating or "grazing" continually.

Sometimes hunger and thirst signals get confused and a person snacks on something to eat when they are actually thirsty and not hungry; it would be better to have a thirst quenching snack. This happens particularly to active people, so before you snack, think about whether you are hungry or thirsty. There are lots of foods and drinks to snack on that have the bonus of energy plus nutrients for action! See appendix D for over 50 suggestions that will suit your snacking mood whether it be thirsty, smooth, crunchy, juicy, fun, or really hungry. So, "nosh" away!

Supplements

Many people regularly take vitamin and mineral supplements, often in very large doses. With the possible exception of iron or calcium, active women do not need to take vitamin and mineral supplements. Your requirements for only four vitamins increase with being very active: thiamine, niacin, riboflavin, and pantothenic acid; they are abundant in our food supply. Vitamin pills do not give you any—let alone MORE— energy and they cannot replace eating "real" food for your energy and nutrient needs.

It is important to consider that nothing is metabolized all on its own; everything you ingest can affect another nutrient or process. The greater the dose of what you take, the greater the probability that it will interfere with something else. These processes are extremely complex and not well understood. Too much of any vitamin can be dangerous and even fatal. Think about all the ways you can be healthy and take care of yourself without popping another pill to "fix it." If you choose to take a supplement, select a multi-vitamin/mineral supplement that does not exceed the Recommended Dietary Allowances of any nutrient.

Water

Last, but by far not the least, is the nutrient water. Probably the most forgotten nutrient of all and yet ignoring it has the most potential for harm. We can live much longer without food than we can without water. It is important to drink before you are thirsty since the osmoreceptors in your brain don't let you know immediately when you need water. When you are losing water and are even mildly dehydrated you might experience fatigue and irritability. Dried lips are the first physical sign of needing water. Many people seldom drink just water. If the thought of plain, old drinking water doesn't sound very appealing, add a drop or two of lemon juice to liven it up or burst into some fizzy mineral water. You need at least six to eight cups of clear liquid each day and more when you are active—add two cups for every one hour of aerobic exercise. Be sure a portion of it is water. Make water one of your everyday health kicks!

Some of these recommendations may not sound like what you had been taught years ago, or what you remember reading. Sensational fad diets often grabbed the headlines and filled magazines distorting good nutritional practice which generally emphasized selecting a variety of foods from the basic food groups. This history has been unfortunate and has contributed to misinformation and much confusion. Today, much is still unknown, but more attention is being paid to scientifically substantiated nutritional information being presented by trained nutritionists.

When you decide that dietary changes need to be made, just as with incorporating physical activity into your life, make those changes one small step at a time. With the combination of nurturing your body with good food choices and activity you, too, can be an energetic woman. Each simple change will make an impact toward the attrACTIVE you.

Recommended Reading

Jane Brody's Nutrition Book, Jane Brody. Bantam Books, New York, NY., 1986.
American Dietetic Association Family Cookbook. Prentice Hall Press, New York, NY., 1987.

5

Living With Stress

don't overdo it.
underdo it.
you aren't running because
you're in a hurry to get somewhere

Fred Rohé

So much has been written about stress; stress workshops and manuals abound. And it's no wonder. Statistically, stress has a very poor reputation when it comes to disease and hospitalizations. Stress related diseases are taken seriously in the medical world. Included in this category are: several kinds of heart diseases, hypertension, many gastrointestinal and pulmonary disorders, and numerous skin conditions. The list goes on and on. And stress is the culprit.

A more careful look into the issue of stress reveals that there is both positive and negative stress and either can cause health problems. Therefore, *how we choose* to handle stress is the most important health factor . . . not a total elimination of stress from our lives. How boring and flat that would be! Just think: no sports (they are certainly stressful for players and spectators), no theater (stage fright would prohibit it), no "falling in love" . . . probably the most stressful of all human activity.

We're not ready to give up stress (even if we could)—good stress (eustress) or bad stress (distress). What we think is important is to be able to:

- recognize stress and its origins
- develop tools for responding to it
- be conscious of dealing with it

- have a sense of being in charge of it, rather than the other way around, so that there is a possibility of it being a catalyst for life and creativity.

Admittedly this is the ideal. Minimally, our goal is to ward off harmful effects of stress.

SIGNS OF STRESS

Our minds, bodies, and spirits clearly let us know when we are stressed. The trick is learning to pick up the signals—only then can we do anything to change the responses to stress. For example, our brains let us know we are overloaded when we don't think as clearly. We are more easily distracted and not so sharp. We hear ourselves saying, "I just can't think," or, "I can't seem to remember anything." Some of us, instead of functioning in low gear, run our brains in very high gear when we are stressed . . . this manic brain state cannot be maintained for long. In this stressed mental state we can no longer make decisions, certainly not the same level of decisions made when our minds are not stressed and are rested. Please note that eustress, or positive stress, has the same effect on our brains, bodies, and spirits as distress. Physiologically the processes are the same. This means that getting that "A +," promotion, vacation, etc., can rev up or slow down the mind just as much as loss, acute anger, or a bout with the flu.

When we are stressed we will notice emotional changes too, i.e., crying unexpectedly, angry outbursts, lack of trust, overreacting, or withdrawing and giving little or no reaction to situations and people. We might feel anxious or depressed; our self-esteem will be down.

At the same time, our bodies (which are also part of the phenomena mentioned above) will signal us with headaches, sweaty palms, lower back pain, rashes, stomach aches, a rapid pulse . . . on and on go the signals. Sometimes we notice a whole combination of physical alarms (dry mouth, tight neck muscles, "funny feeling" in my stomach). Each one of us has experienced these warning signals; most can be summed up as changes in our bodies and minds: changes in sleep patterns (sleeping more, sleeping less), changes in eating (overeating, loss of appetite), changes in strength (usually a feeling of weakness).

Our spirits are not so alive when we are distressed. We speak of feeling "down" and "spiritless." When we are eustressed we soar . . . but we can't soar forever. Spiritual soaring is still experienced by our bodies as stressful and in need of attention and eventually some rest is needed for balance. In societies where "if a little is good, more must be better" it is hard to accept the fact that "more" spiritual insight, mediation, or altered state can be stressful. But there is such a thing as being spiritually greedy—it is not often addressed as a problem. Striving for and achieving spiritual enlightenment, perfection, heights (different religions describe it differently) can reach unhealthy stress levels. No religion is exempt from this hazard. It is a problem spiritually, just as it is an emotional and physical hazard. Balance is needed.

These are our signs—a coordinated effort of our total self; these signs are multiple and clear because they need to be. We must be able to recognize stress and respond appropriately. In ancient times humans responded with "fight or flight" so that they could survive physical danger. The dangers which threaten us today are no less serious. In a very real sense the issue is still survival . . . mental, emotional, and spiritual survival as well as physical survival. And beyond mere survival is health and well-being.

IDENTIFYING THE SOURCES OF STRESS

Quite simple the sources of stress are people (including ourselves), places, and things. Some we can change or modify and others we cannot. It is critical that we discover which we can, which we cannot and then decide what we will do. Let's look at people first.

People at Work

Whom do I experience as a stressor?
_____ boss
_____ co-worker
_____ administrators
_____ occasional workers
_____ people who answer to me or look to me for guidance

- Are their expectations different from mine?
- Are their personalities very different?
- Their values? Their biological clocks (they value early morning meetings, early morning output . . . or late)?
- Do they have annoying habits?

Ask:

- How stressful are they? (on a scale of 1-10)
- Can I avoid them?
- Can I modify my work pattern so that I have less contact?
- Can I communicate with them differently? (more directly, less directly, in writing, on the telephone, with others, alone?)

To just *endure* a person at work can add to the stress. To be working on a difficult relationship can often help. Problem solving with yourself alone (writing down possibilities and then assessing them) or with a trusted friend, or even with the person who is a stressor, can all be part of a plan to deal with work-person stress.

People at Home

Again, be specific. Who are they?

_____ spouse or partner
_____ parent
_____ relative
_____ child
_____ pet (we prefer to consider pets as at-home people)
_____ combinations of any of the above (especially on holidays and special occasions)

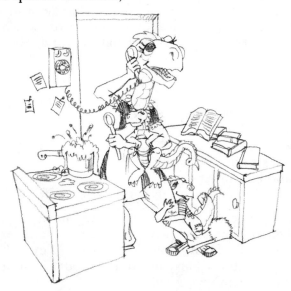

Ask yourself the same kinds of specific questions as those used for assessing the work situation and personalities there. Be specific in pinpointing the stressful ones and stressful situations. Often the situations can be avoided when the people cannot. For example, if visits with in-laws are high-risk times of stress, consider shorter visits and/or less frequent visits. Have a specific idea of what you will do together or separately. Have you thought about separate vacations? Once in a while? Or sometimes separate from _____ (children, family, friends, spouse)?

Varying ways of communicating can also be helpful in family situations. Careful picking of time for important conversations, attention to place and words chosen, and developing listening skills can be important tools for dealing with stress in intimate relationships. (More in chapter 6.)

People in the Community

Community is a broad term meant to include people in your city or neighborhood, city, school, and state organizations, national government, church, synagogue, or religious groups. If you are a person who is involved in issues about which you are committed and feel strongly, there is bound to be tension and stress. Ask yourself: Am I spread too thin? Do too many issues and people seem to demand my attention? Which are most important? What are my priorities? How will I spend that portion of my life energy I designate as "global" (anything outside of my immediate daily living)?

There are so many people, so many meetings, so many decisions linked to being an active person in a community. All important issues cannot be resolved by us, in our time frame, according to our style. The stress of being a caring or concerned citizen can be very great and take a heavy toll. And if I am torn by stress, I will not be very creative and available to others . . . which is what stimulated the care in the first place!

Places and Things

Besides people as sources of stress there are locations—geographies if you will—which in themselves are stressful. Cities, work space, living space, communal space do effect our well-being. How do each effect our senses? What is the noise level? How do they look? Smell? Are they crowded, dark, too bright? Dangerous? Too hot? Cold? What can I do to change or modify them?

Finally, consider things or factors. Cars, machines, objects of any sort (so-called art pieces), music, foods, transportation. Your list will vary depending on whether you are an urban or rural person, what part of the country you live in, what you do all day, what you do on vacations. Danger is a stress factor. Happiness and success are stress factors. "Things" may be very abstract or concrete, but they do need some attention in an assessment of "Where's the stress?"

WHAT CAN I DO ABOUT STRESS?

Looking over the previous paragraphs, one thing becomes clear. Change is a cause of stress. Any change. Good things happen. Bad things happen. Both are change and produce stress. Change is not good or bad—it is inevitable! There is no sense in trying to eliminate the cause; our response to change is what matters.

Most of this program is directed at using our bodies in motion—specifically aerobically—as a way of and towards health. We consider using aerobic activity three to five times per week as a primary tool for preventing an unhealthy build-up of stress and a tool for dealing with stress. Instead of yelling at a co-worker, child, or partner, or kicking the dog . . . go for a long hard walk or a fast bike ride. Or, at least do these things before making a decision when pressures have built up. Besides the physical effects of the activity, you are giving yourself some valuable think time. Aerobic activity does not make stress go away but it can:

- improve sleep patterns (so that we are rested enough to figure out how to deal with this particularly stressing situation)
- reduce how much it "gets us" or we "buy into it"
- put us in touch with "I have choices here," "I am in charge here"
- prevent build up of stress over time (day, week)
- gives us that "think time"
- increase our sense of strength (self-confidence) and ability to respond to the stress or handle it
- promote physical independence (prompting assertive actions)
- release energy for living

But, as dedicated to aerobic activity as we are, we do want to point out other ways of dealing with stress which can be used before the fact (preventively) or after. Among them are:

- MEDITATION which elicits the relaxation response
- BEAUTY, i.e., art, music, nature, poetry, literature
- SOLITUDE
- FRIENDSHIPS, for love and nurturance
- HUMOR to relieve tension and shift perspective

Meditation There are tapes available which are very effective in helping you relax. Relaxing is an identifiable physiological state which can be achieved through the mind. Dr. Herbert Benson *(The Relaxation Response)* has researched this phenomenon and written extensively about it. We recommend the use of tapes, certainly when beginning meditation, because it is easier to follow another's voice, rather than try to remember the next step or phrase. Basically, what is involved is first breathing in a slow, patterned way, then relaxing one's muscles and freeing one's mind. Slow breathing can be done by taking in a breath to the count of five, holding it for five counts and releasing it to the count of five. The latter can be done by concentration on a phrase or sound or an image. Putting the mind at rest for 5 to 30 minutes, IN COMBINATION with the body, is a marvelous tool for responding to stress. For more relaxation techniques see appendix F.

Sometimes we find women "turned off" to meditation or uncomfortable with it because it seems to them to be for another "type" of woman . . . images of placid, stoic, "airy." Not necessarily true. There is no particular "type" suited for meditation. Meditation is not necessarily limited to 20 or 30 minutes in length. You can be a "closet meditator." Slip away—to the women's room if convenient and quiet–and take five minutes to breath slowly, relax, and imagine yourself on a warm—not hot—beach, or in a cool, sunny meadow. In your mind listen to the beautiful sounds, smell the air, feel the breeze, touch the earth. Be there. Be refreshed. Then decide to leave this place in your mind and return to the job, the kids, Uncle Ralph, or the bill collectors. Meditating is no big deal. It's just a convenient, helpful tool. Like aerobic exercise, it is not a panacea.

Beauty The Navajo Blessing Way advises us to "Walk in Beauty." Look for it and go with it. Beauty is a powerful, available tool for dealing with stress.

CATHARINE I remember talking with a young, concerned—and stressed—doctor in the parking lot of our hospital one early winter evening shortly after five. Suddenly, my eye caught sight of the mountains as the sun was setting. We both stopped what we were doing and truly enjoyed the three minutes of dramatic beauty played out before us. Costing us nothing but three minutes of attention and giving back a sigh, a moment of rest and refreshment.

• • •

Not all of us have mountains to look at, but all can get in touch with beauty. Stop at a florist shop and look, smell, enjoy. A song takes from 2 to 30 minutes. Pick one and really listen, not as background noise for our day, but as a moment of beauty in itself.

As Navajos say:
> *with beauty before you, go*
> *with beauty above you, go*
> *with beauty beside you, go*
> *with beauty behind you, go*
> *with beauty all around you, go.*

But first you must seek it out and pay attention.

Solitude First we must believe that we can be only with ourselves and that we are worthwhile company. This too is something which takes time and experience. We have discovered valuable solitude in running and swimming. This is MY TIME. Besides activity time alone, time alone with my thoughts, sitting quietly inside or outside, or strolling with no specific destination can be valuable and a good preventive resource in relationship to stress therapy.

Friends and Humor Friends are sources of understanding and support in all seasons of life. Being understood AS WE ARE is a great antidote for stress. With friends we can talk through feelings and thoughts, they can be a release valve, a sounding board, a source of advice. They are like no other—not even partners. There are different friends for different moments in our lives. Sometimes they are part of our stress tool called "humor"; they help us laugh at ourselves, our situations, our responses. They help us see life differently. But our friends are not the only source of humor: books, T.V., people on the street, or in performance make us LAUGH . . . a great physical exercise in itself! Here too the endorphines are released and we experience a real biochemical change. And we are refreshed and renewed. Norman Cousins, who has written and lectured about the therapeutic effects of laughter, is careful to point out that it is not a cure, but a powerful and helpful response to pain, illness, in short, stress. It is not the only or always appropriate response called for, but, what fun it is when we use it. The child is alive and well. We are alive and balanced for a time. We see life a little differently; our perspective changes and we are changed. From this new point of view, we can be the directors, rather than the victims of stress.

Humor will be a most welcome helpmate when undertaking the eight week (lifetime?) program of attrACTIVE Woman. Getting physical can be very funny at times. Our "beginner's mistake," our "goofs" along the way, can bring a smile to ourselves and others. Trips, slips, and pratfalls are the stuff of Laurel and Hardy . . . and a lot of us. (We're not talking about pain and getting hurt, only those ungraceful movements when we find ourselves learning, being OK children again). Humor says to us: hey, don't expect to be an expert right away; give yourself time to develop skill and control.

CATHARINE If I didn't have a sense of humor, I'd never have survived so many times coming in last! I'd never have learned to fix a flat tire, get up from a fall, or reach the top of the mountain.

• • •

Stress. Friend or foe? You decide. A lot of the quality of your life depends on it.

Recommended Reading

StressMap: Essi System's Self-Scoring Questionnaire and Action Planning Guide— Personal Diary Edition, Esther M. Orioli, M.S., and Dennis T. Jaffe, Ph.D. Copyright 1987. Newmarket Press, 18 East 48 Street, New York, NY 10017.
The Stress of Life, Hans Selye. McGraw-Hill, New York, 1978.
Codependent No More, Melody Beattie. Harper & Row/Hazelden, San Francisco, CA, 1988.

6

Emotions: High, Low, and Everything in Between

... damn everything that won't get into the circle,
that won't enjoy,
that won't throw its heart into the tension,
surprise, fear and delight
of the circus,
the round world,
the full existence ...

S. Helen Kelley

We can't write a book about mental health without talking about emotions. After all, when we're asked, "How do you feel?" we aren't limited in our response to describing something physical; we often respond by naming an emotion. "I feel sad." Or happy, angry, anxious, guilty, excited, ... in love. Strong, powerful stuff. The stuff of life.

Emotions are like the seasonings of life. We have a lot of different kinds. Some are strong and only a pinch is needed on a certain day. On another, a lot more is needed to bring out the true flavor of our reality. Any less, and the moment is somehow not "right"—it's flatter than our reality. Emotions are not in charge of "what kind" and "how much"—I am the one in charge ... I do not have to be the victim of my emotions. I only have to recognize their presence and express them appropriately. Sometimes that's a tall order. But we have noticed that the healthiest women we know and with whom we work are those who are in touch with their feelings—all of them. Women who don't put their energy into denying feelings, but rather into learning about them and figuring out how they can own them and express them without harming themselves or others.

Like seasonings, no emotions are bad—they just need to be used in different amounts at different times with different people. They are part of our reality; they bring out and highlight moments. Often we remember an event because of the emotional content or context and intensity.

CLEAR THINKING—CLEAR FEELING

In order to identify emotions and give them direction we first need to distinguish them from thoughts. Listen:

"I feel that is incorrect."
"I feel the idea is not sound."
"I feel Mary Smith would be a good president."
"I feel you are wrong."
"I feel you are full of _____!"

In each case feeling is *not* what is going on. Thinking is. Try it on. "I think that is incorrect," "I think you are wrong," "I think she would be a good president." Distinguish the process. Somehow many of us have gotten the idea that to say "I feel" is "softer" or more acceptable than to clearly say "I think"—or maybe it is a surprise to some that women *do* think, not just feel! Claim that thinking power and use it. The two activities are not mutually exclusive. Personality inventories (especially the Myers-Briggs) show that some people feel first and think a bit later; others start thinking in response to an event or remark and then get in touch with their feelings flowing from it. Neither is a "better" way of responding. Women and men, as such, do not differ in this regard. Some women feel first; some men feel first. Some women start thinking first, some men start thinking first. We have noticed, however, that there is a societal stereotype which assumes that women feel first (last, and always) and that men are the thinkers who sort of save us from "emotional" (or hysterical) women. We don't buy that and research doesn't support it either. It is the same societal stereotyping that assumes men are emotionally inept and can only think. This kind of short-sighted thinking leaves no room for growth for women or men. For many there is a habit of speaking in the "I feel" mode. Habits are hard to break; this one can be broken by a slight pause before speaking to decide, "What's going on here? Feeling? Or thinking?"

Associated with this is figuring out if the other person is "feeling" or "thinking" when they say, "I feel. . . . " Being confused between the two activities just muddies things up, and emotions are too important for that. Clear thinking and clear feeling are both part of becoming attrACTIVE. When you are unclear whether a person is thinking or feeling, simply "check in" with them by asking.

Get In Touch—Specifically

After distinguishing what's going on, the next step is to identify which emotion we are feeling. There can be confusion here too. Partly this is because many think some emotions are negative and no one wants to be feeling one of the unacceptable ones. So I will say, "I'm hurt," when "I'm angry" is more accurate. Or tears will stream and one thinks: "she's sad" because to think of her as raging is "not nice." (When I am the one raging it can be scary to me to realize this; to think of myself as "hurt" or "sad" is more acceptable, but it is not more accurate.) The fact is, there *are* tears of angry frustration. They need to be recognized for what they are: not sadness, not weakness, but strong, energy-filled ANGRY tears.

Anger is a difficult emotion for many women to own. Yet to deny it denies a part of our human energy. It is powerful. It can be creative. If no one got angry, there would be very little change. Little justice. Little energy put into cures for cancer or muscular dystrophy. We raise money for research in these areas because we are angry at the loss of life, the limitations of living, the unfairness of it all. Pictures are painted, poetry written, songs sung out of feelings of anger. Feelings with which the artist is in touch, and willing and able to express. We listen, we look, we read, and we can say: "I recognize that. It is true. I have felt just like that too." How beautifully human. How important.

So many emotions, such variety. Such nuance. There isn't just *angry* but *enraged, annoyed, grumpy, irritated, steaming, seething.* There isn't just *happy,* there is *delighted, glad, joyful, ecstatic.* And none of them are *good* or *bad,* they simply are—feelings. We urge you to get in touch—specifically.

To go into the topic of emotions, women, and well-being in depth would take a whole book (and has already been done very well by professionals in the area of psychology). But a few words are called for to address emotions which are suppressed, which seem to interfere with women pursuing their active, healthy lives.

Bottling Up Feelings Can Be Unhealthy

In our groups, women mention feelings of guilt, embarrassment, fear, depression, and anger as stumbling blocks to daily living and health. These feelings frequently act as barriers to their goals. We hear a lot of, "So, what can I do about them?" as if getting rid of the feelings would be in order. This is much different from "So, what can I do?" which accepts both responsibility and the option of control. When women want to rid themselves of feelings it often leads to stuffing the feelings away rather than owning them and dealing with them now, or at an appropriate time. Suppressing emotions (or pretending we don't have them) is part of the profile of stress discussed in chapter 5. And suppressed emotions seem to build up and take on a whole new power inside that "eats" away at us. When they are strong enough, they have a sneaky way of getting out anyway, something like a time bomb exploding. Sometimes the explosion is in the form of anger which seems disproportionate to the situation (like the proverbial straw that breaks the camel's back). Suppressed fear or anger that doesn't take the form of an explosion often creeps out in the form of a headache or back pain. Anxiety may take the disguise of hives or fever blisters. The list of physical symptoms or signs could go on and on and they have their roots in strong emotions. Bottling up feelings simply does not work—it can be very unhealthy for all concerned.

We also think that women who would do away with these difficult emotions probably have not had to deal with persons who have "a flat affect" which means virtually no ability to feel emotions or express them. This disability is a characteristic of some mental disorders and is a terrible handicap.

On the other hand, "What can I do?" is a statement recognizing that I am not the victim of my feelings of guilt, anger, or depression, but rather I am in charge of my feelings and my life. I'm ready for the sometimes difficult task of making decisions about my feelings. I recognize I can do many things. I have choices. It is very important to recognize this. Do a little brain-storming. For instance:

Guilt

"I could feel more guilty."
(do I really want to?)
"I could feel no guilt."

(probably unrealistic)
"I could feel 10 percent guilty."
(more possible)
"I could remind myself that guilt is just a feeling."
(good move)
"I could think about guilt being OK and normal and that I don't have only guilty feelings; maybe there are some other feelings here too."
(this kind of expanding and searching out more than surface feelings can be very helpful and self-informing)

Can you imagine the sense of freedom for some women when they recognize that guilt is an option? That they don't have to "do guilt"! Or they won't have to write out an emotional blank check payable in any amount?

Feeling quilty also makes it difficult to be assertive. When overwhelmed by guilt, a person is more likely to either withdraw, or be aggressive. Both are very limited responses.

Taking time with guilt allows for a sense of responsibility. When we no longer are into the game of blaming someone else with "you make me feel so guilty," we are better able to make healthy decisions for ourselves.

This kind of getting in touch with a feeling and thinking about it can be used with other "difficult" feelings (like fear, jealousy, depression, anger). It is helpful because it reminds us that we can make decisions about feelings. Not whether we have them or not, but how much attention or energy to put into them and how to express them. The latter is critical.

Anger
"I'll kill the . . . ."
  (not practical, considering the consequences)
"I am feeling the anger; it is hot; I'll take it (me) for a walk."
  (good classic decision)
"I'm feeling so angry; this is a good time to tell him about it."
  (other options: writing him, picking another time, another place—but not stuffing it)
"I'll eat the leftover pie."
  (short-term pleasure; does nothing to get the anger expressed . . . we know, we've both tried it!)

Other options:
— *stewing* all day and polluting other activities with our anger
— talking about it with others
— discussing my possible responses with a friend
— pounding a pillow
— stuffing the feeling away
— pouting
— writing in my journal
— sleeping

There are lots of choices. And you can pick one. NOT to choose is to choose . . . to choose to let *anything* happen with my anger. It's writing that emotional blank check—and as dangerous as writing a financial blank check! Few of us would do that.

Depression

Everyone, at one time or another, feels "depressed"—that's normal, a part of the human condition. But there is another kind of depression which isn't normal and needs professional help and sometimes medication. If you are concerned about your depression, please consult with your physician or mental health professional, because this kind of clinical depression can be treated.

What's particularly difficult about any type of depression, is that when you're feeling it, it is hard to remember you ever felt good. It's hard to think, period. So don't try to think when you're depressed. Think ahead. If you are one who knows that this is a rather frequent and difficult emotion to handle, take time when you're feeling like yourself to write down what is helpful. For instance, make three lists:

PEOPLE:
When I'm with _____ I feel good about myself.
When I talk to _____ on the telephone I feel good about myself.
I enjoy writing to _____ .

PLACES:
When I am _____ (i.e., in the park, my garden, in the chapel, the museum) I feel good about myself.
When I am in _____ (i.e., San Francisco, Spain, etc.) I feel good.

When I am _____ (think of your own special place),
I feel good.

THINGS:
When I _____ (ride my bike, swim, run) I feel good.
When I _____ (read, shop, talk, bake bread) I feel
good about myself.

Make your lists very specific and very personal. List who and
what works for you. And add to the list, keep it handy so that
when the "blahs" and "blues" hit you don't have to think, you
only have to choose. Some of the items may be readily available,
like looking at picture books, or other things which connect you
to that "good space," that good image. Some might take planning, such as, getting to Spain or San Francisco.

There are excellent tapes on the market which guide one's
imagination and allow you to "be" somewhere pleasant, somewhere inside yourself (it's *your* imagination remember, it's
only being guided by another) where you can connect with

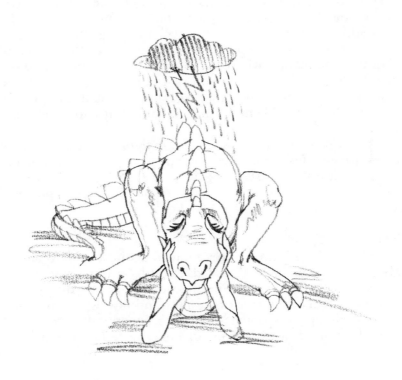

"good" energy and positive feelings about yourself. Ocean sounds, the tide rolling in, over and over, might offer you that place.

One technique for expressing some of these difficult emotions is this statement:

"I feel _____ when you _____ because _____ ."

This facilitates clarity. It allows you to identify your feeling, own it, and communicate it to another in a straightforward manner without blaming anyone. It is so much better than using "You make me feel so _____ !" With this statement the other person is immediately on the defense because they are being blamed or feel attacked and they probably do not know why or what happened. The "reach out" statement gives the other person a chance to learn exactly which feeling you have and to consider how they are involved. This does not mean that your emotions will automatically have the power to stop behavior; it simply keeps the communication clear and straight.

How different all of this is from saying "she made me feel guilty," or "he made me so mad," or "they made me feel depressed." No one can make you feel anything. Impossible. "I feel" puts the ownership where it belongs, and the power of choice in the matter, where it belongs. "They"—out there—is not the location of the emotion or the decision. attrACTIVE women are women in the process of discovering this important fact. It eliminates blaming and reclaims self-knowledge and power.

Using this kind of statement doesn't come automatically, it takes a conscious effort and it helps to practice saying it out loud to yourself at first. You might be surprised at the results this handy tool can offer in your professional as well as personal life.

Sex

So far in this book we haven't talked about sex. We've talked about being women and that does address our primary sexuality—our total way of being the women we are. But sex and how we feel about ourselves sexually and how we express ourselves sexually is a specific area which needs attention.

To be honest, it is difficult to find the right chapter for a

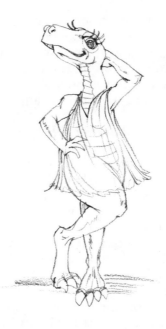

discussion of sex. Surely it fits into a chapter on psychology and certainly in one on physiology. But we have decided to put it in this chapter on emotions partly because it is such an emotional topic, but mostly because we so often talk about "feeling sexy" or having "sexual" feelings.

Again—and we don't want to belabor the topic—these are feelings: not good or bad. Simply, feelings. How we choose to act upon them may be judged by ourselves as good or bad, appropriate, or inappropriate. But the feelings are OK. So the first step towards healthy sexuality is accepting the feelings as OK; the next step is accepting our bodies.

Here there seems to be difficulty and two extremes become apparent.

1. I don't accept my body; it is all wrong. I can't be sexy or feel sexual until my body is "right" (perfect; looks like _____).

2. I know I am "sexy" if *he* (or *she*) tells me so.

Either point of view is a flashing yellow light. Dangerous. Watch out. If you are continually putting down your body, it is virtually impossible to let it send you "sexy" signals because when it does, you deny them. "I can't be feeling this way because I'm not beautiful." This is a two-way put-down. It puts down the one who is sending the signals ("what poor taste he has to send such a message") and it puts down yourself as one unworthy of this attention. This isn't healthy . . . and it's no fun, either!

On the other end of the unhealthy scale is the woman who is constantly seeking body-validation sexually. "Once is not enough" . . . nor a hundred times. Body insecurity is tied up with sex and sex cannot provide body security. It is not fair to your partner or yourself. We are not saying that having someone make love to us and making love to another is a sign of insecurity. Making love is a sign of a healthy sexuality. What is questionable is when a woman depends solely on sex for validation of her body . . . constantly needing another to validate herself through sex.

Sometimes in our groups women have said something like this: "My husband wants me to lose weight. If I don't, I'll lose him." There is fear and almost panic behind such a statement because it is a statement of what the woman has feared for most of her life and society has reinforced. But the statement needs to be looked at from a few different perspectives.

The first consideration is her image of what is "sexy" and attractive. What is it that she lacks physically which would warrant being deprived of sexual intimacy? What is the range in height, weight, size, shape into which she must fit herself in order to qualify for female beauty or sexual attractiveness? Next, what is his image of what is "sexy" and attractive? There have been "attractiveness" tests given to men and women. The findings reveal that within the heterosexual population the range of acceptable body size and type for women is more narrowly perceived by women than by men! What we think they want, isn't necessarily so! As one young man said recently, "They all look good to me!" And this was a young man; generally, as men get older and more experienced, they discover the delightful varieties of beautiful women. Their previous immature tastes, also reinforced by society's fantasies, have been replaced by a more satisfying reality than that offered by advertisements. Both women and men, or perhaps more accurately, girls and boys, buy into images of women which are not based on what is found to be really sexually attractive by adults.

Yet the expectations hang on and cause pain to both women and men. Time and again we hear people talking about "sexy" or attractive women and time and again we hear a confirmation that beauty IS in the eye of the beholder . . . not fashion makers who are merely out to sell clothes.

Take time out to think about someone whom you consider to be beautiful yet who doesn't fit the North American stereotype. Most of us do know women who differ from the "cover girl" image. Women who are attractive, vital, charming, interesting . . . *and* sexy.

Often it is a woman's perception that she is only sexually attractive at a certain weight and shape and she believes that is what her partner wants also. But what if a partner clearly states: "To be attractive to me sexually, you must become slim." We cannot presume to give a glib answer. This is a very difficult situation and may be a dilemma. Only an individual couple will be able to determine what to do. We hope that decisions about what to do would be based on more than that cold statement which sounds like an ultimatum. As a way of reaching a decision, we would recommend couple counseling in order to more thoroughly explore underlying fears and/or expectations of both partners. It may prove to be insurmountable; it is more likely that this type of statement cloaks other issues. If you are serious about sex, you'll check it out rather than comply without consent and risk feeling sexually unsure of your body.

What we are saying is that when it comes to sex and feeling sexual, it is not our bodies that need changing so much as our minds. When we are at war with our bodies we are usually also at war with our sexuality. Frigidity and promiscuity are battle signals.

ACTIVE AND SEXUALLY HEALTHY

MARVEL In working with women suffering from disordered eating I have seen both ends of the spectrum. For some women the thought of anyone seeing their bodies, much less touching it sends them into a panic and utter terror. There is no option for lovemaking or sharing physical intimacies for these women in their present state. On the other extreme are women who end up having sex with many partners, "one night stands," a promiscuous attempt to accept their bodies. The thought (or the subconscious thought) goes something like this: "If someone wants to have sex with me, obviously I must be attractive or sexy or beautiful or OK." Of course this thinking backfires and, following the encounter, she hates herself, feels repulsed by what she has done, and then the thoughts are something like, "I was right all the time, I am an ugly, no good tramp." So her "ugly" self-thoughts are reinforced over and over again. It is a vicious circle downward as long as she is depending on sex and another person for her validation. Either extreme is devastating and the woman misses out on self-esteem and growth. She sees herself as unattractive and gets dangerously stuck there.

• • •

In her long overdue book, *How to Make Love to the Same Person for the Rest of Your Life,* Dagmar O'Connor makes a strong case for the connection between being active and being sexually healthy.

Staying in shape physically is a prime way we can stay in shape sexually. By walking, jogging, skiing, playing tennis, or swimming together, we get our hearts beating, our blood flowing, and our "juices" going again. We feel more vital and more sensitive, stronger and less prone to fatigue, and ultimately, we feel more relaxed. Just the smallest regular regimen of exercise can diminish physical tension and emotional stress immeasurably, leaving us both more willing and more able to enjoy ourselves sexually. Recently, volumes have been written about the joys of jogging—physical fitness is enjoying an unprecedented vogue—so I will not go on ad nauseam about the general benefits of getting in shape. But it is worth stressing that sex, first and foremost, is a PHYSICAL ACT: We simply cannot get sexual until we get physical.

We would not stress participating in activities together as a necessary part of the physical activities and their connection with being sexual, but physical activities can be fun to share.

It might surprise you how interconnected being active and being attractive are.

MARVEL I can't remember feeling more appealing and satisfied about my looks than in a statewide triathlon. I was doing

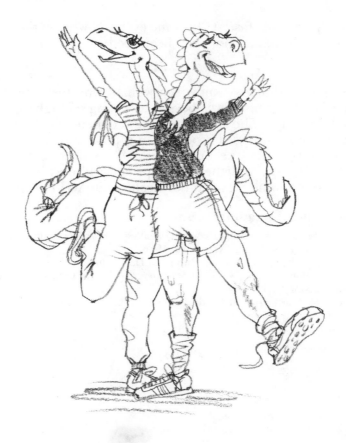

the running leg which was 10 kilometers and somehow being part of a team was especially inspiring to me that crisp fall day. My adrenaline was high and I started out fast, pulling away from the cheering crowds at the exchange sight. At the first bend of the downhill section I was stretching out, barely aware of the pavement beneath my feet and feeling strong when my friend (and greatest supporter!) cupped his hands around his mouth and shouted with all the power and love one man could muster "YOU'RE BEAUTIFUL!" I soared . . . my body and soul united in a thrill of exhilaration. I have never felt more beautiful in my entire life. Sometimes I close my eyes, take a deep breath and relive that sensation . . . that moment of thorough and sensual beauty that is mine to treasure forever! (Incidentally I ran my fastest 10K time ever and we won the triathlon for which we had not even been seeded!)

• • •

The sexiest thing we know is a woman who feels and looks confident. She experiences herself as strong enough and wise enough for living. She is not fragile and dependent on another to "make her happy." Through being physically active as we suggest, anyone can be on the way to discovering this sexy attrACTIVE self, and then perhaps she will decide to share herself with another . . . another healthy attrACTIVE person.

Recommended Reading

How To Make Love To the Same Person For the Rest of Your Life, Dagmar O'Connor. Bantam Paperbacks, New York, 1986.

The Angry Book, Theodore Isaac Rubin. M.D. Macmillan, New York, 1969.

Swept Away: Why Women Fear Their Own Sexuality, Carol Cassell. Simon and Schuster, New York, 1984.

The Dance of Anger, Harriet Goldhor Lerner, Ph.D. Harper and Row, New York, 1985.

7

Whole-ly Holy

Be prepared at all times
for the gifts of God
and be ready always
for new ones.
For God is a thousand times
more ready to give
than we are to receive.

Meister Eckhart

For several chapters now we have discussed the interconnectedness of ourselves: body-mind-emotions. Until now spirit,
or the spiritual, has not been addressed. Recently the spiritual
dimensions of a holistic approach to health and well-being are
being discussed in periodicals and an occasional book. We've
waited a long time for this inclusive approach.

The body has been a topic of importance in world religions
for thousands of years. It has been viewed as a stumbling block
to spiritual progress and also as a means to achieving enlightenment. Although an extensive historical review of various
world religions (Buddhism, Islam, Judaism, Hinduism, Chris-
tianity) might be interesting, it will not be the focus of this
chapter.

RELIGIOUS BELIEFS CAN AFFECT BODY IMAGE

Each of us has some kind of religious history, or rootedness;
each of us probably has read about and explored other religious
or metaphysical "paths." What we propose to do is have you
look at both: religious "givens" (or teachings), and new possible
directions for spiritual growth, and do a bit of analyzing or
assessing according to spiritual values.

ASK YOURSELF:

Does my religious heritage focus on body?

_____ at all _____ somewhat _____ certain parts/functions.

Does my tradition give me any information, any messages about _____ my body, or _____ others' bodies?

Is this attitude or information

_____ positive? _____ negative? _____ scary?

Does it promote

_____ ignoring the body? _____ celebrating it? _____ a mixture?

Does it approach the body intellectually?

What kind of mixture do I see in my religious heritage?

Does my spirit today need a positive body image in order to live fully?

How can I enhance my body image with and through religious and/or spiritual practices or beliefs?

We are not suggesting that a particular religious tradition has all the answers. We do think it might be helpful to examine the previous questions in relationship to some of the religions of our time so that you can continue your reflection. Perhaps you will be able to incorporate their insights, our perception of their insights, and your own observations into your own religious or spiritual journey.

Christian

It is amazing to us that women of the same religion can have such different answers to these questions. For example, some Christian women may see the body as a constant burden to be overcome. Dangerous. "An occasion of sin." Something to be disciplined, brought under control of the mind and spirit. After much struggling, a "good Christian" can overcome the body and become more "angelic," more spiritual. Actually, this attitude is pretty insulting to the Creator: we were not created to BE angels, but human beings, and trying to "be like the angels" is setting an impossible course, sure to fail— since we don't know what angels are like or what is expected for their health and happiness. Also, it is a first cousin of the *Be Perfect Syndrome* so familiar to many. Besides being setup for failure, "be perfect" is probably a poor translation of the Greek in John's gospel ("Be perfect as my heavenly Father is perfect"). If you go back to the original Greek root, *telos*, you find that the word means to be complete or to "be fully." In this context, that would be to be fully human, just as "my father" is fully divine. "Be who you are intended to be—fully." What a difference this translation makes! Being "perfect" is impossible for "amateur human beings" (a descriptive phrase from one of our friends), but being as human as possible is within the realm of possibility—and of greater benefit to others. Striving to be perfect can be quite a strain on us and everyone around us.

This "Christian" attitude of separating body and soul actually had its roots in a pre-Christian dualism which perceived the body as evil (and by the way "feminine") and the mind as "pure" spirit (and—you guessed it—"masculine"). The mind was clearly superior to the body. The spiritual goal was to be free of the body. Even bodily functions were avoided, hence these practitioners didn't bathe much. Early Christians held onto some of these beliefs, though none of them were essentially Christian in nature. Holding on to this belief has led some to a distrust and fear of the body. For them, to focus on the physical might mean to "like it too much" and abandoning the intellect—it would mean "living like an animal," or "lower" form of creation. This has not been our experience. When we run or cycle we have a block of time to think and process what we have read and our own and others' thoughts about God and creation. We worship by running, swimming, cycling toward God and with God.

CATHARINE My bike becomes my prayer wheel(s) and my experience—not that of any other creature (fish, flower, person)—but of me, Catharine, daughter of God, child of creation. Uniquely human and exercising not only my mind, but my body as well . . . we do not have to make a choice between one aspect of self or the other. We couldn't even if we tried.

• • •

If one reads the Christian scriptures, and Paul in particular, there is a tradition of acceptance of the body and respect for it. Forty times in the gospels, and forty times in Paul's writings "body" is mentioned—and not as something evil. This is some of what we find:

> *Your body you know is the temple of the Holy Spirit*
> (1Cor. 6:19)
>
> *Worship God . . . by offering your living bodies as a holy sacrifice (a special prayer)*
> (Rom. 12:1)
>
> *Use your body for the glory of God*
> (1Cor. 6:20)
>
> *All a woman need worry about is being holy in body and spirit.*
> (1Cor. 7:34)

And most powerfully
> *Now you are the body of Christ and individually members of it.*
> (1Cor. 12:27)

Now if Paul had a very negative view of the body he would never have picked that metaphor for Christ!

From being a Jew, Paul had a *basar* (see chapter 1) mentality. That is, an interconnected mentality. Being also very involved in the Greco world, he would have been influenced by their very positive (almost too positive?) regard for the body and its importance. It's hard to find in his writings a negative regard for body. It IS possible to find a concern for balance. Surely, in the gospels and in Paul's writing we find cautions against "worshiping" the body or living only for its glorification. Nowhere do we find it presented as something evil or contrary to God's plan of salvation.

In John's gospel we read of Jesus saying "I came to bring life and bring it abundantly." As Christians we can't imagine that one could experience abundant life and ignore—much less be at war with—one's body. One's precious "temple" of God's Living Spirit.

Let's look at this whole concept of temple. What is a temple for? How is it treated? What do you do in temples? How do you desecrate (make unholy) a temple? A temple is a sacred space wherein one is open to grace, new life, wonder, wisdom. It is a space of encountering the living God. The Jewish temple of old, Christian churches today, Hindu and Buddhist temples—all incorporate aspects or emphasize aspects of this definition. If our bodies are temples, what are the implications? They are sacred space; they are places of meeting God; they can reveal wisdom and wonder; they reveal new life to us and others. In the chapter on nutrition we addressed problems such as tearing down the temples of our bodies by dieting, purging, using abusive drugs, laxatives, etc. Our concern is not only a concern for the physical; if we tear down the temple, where will we worship?

Christian spirituality calls for endurance, truth, and self-awareness. The body can be a spiritual guide in these endeavors. It can show us what is needed to endure—as Paul reflects, to "run the good race":

- having clear priorities
- persisting in the face of trials and difficulties
- accepting temporary setbacks
- respecting my strengths and relying on them and on God as a source of my strength
- accepting my limitations
- forgiving myself for failures
- experiencing joy and love

How can I call myself involved with a God-quest if I know nothing of joy?

Buddhism

Our bodies are full of life. Divine life, our life. Buddhism expresses a very special reverence for life. In his *Asian Journal* Thomas Merton refers to Gary Snyder, poet and Zen theologian, who says that Zen and Tibetan Buddhism are closer than any other schools in Buddhism, but that their methods are in reverse of each other. Zen goes directly to the ground of consciousness and then comes up, exploring other realms of mind, having seen the ground first. Tibetan Buddhism goes down gradually, until the ground of consciousness is reached. That puts it very succinctly—perhaps too succinctly—but clearly makes the point that neither disregards, nor "puts down" the body and our bodily experience.

In 1974 Fred Rohé wrote *The Zen of Running*. In lovely poetry and poetic photography he conveys his experience of Zen meditation through running—running is his "ground;" running for him has become his meditation space. Through it he practices his Zen beliefs:

— be here now, in this moment
— respect your unique "being in the light"
— attend to joy
— use self-discipline as a road to wisdom
— incorporate balance and rhythm in living
— live simply and freely
— be involved in self-creation

For Rohé the smallest moment can contain a whole world of wisdom. It can be a spiritual microcosm.

Zen is like a big sign that says "pay attention: be alert; be in the moment." It asks a consciousness of now: of breath, heart, legs, of temperature, all sensations. If you are in the process of incorporating aspects of the Zen tradition into your spiritual life, perhaps you can be writing (or noticing) your own Zen of Cycling, Zen of Swimming, Zen of Walking. It can become a primary prayer form or an important adjunct to your prayer life. Ancients and moderns have learned that prayer is not limited only to words, or thoughts. It can—perhaps must—be kinesthetic, communal, and perhaps only a way of saying "thank you" for creation. Creation includes yourself.

MARVEL There is no time when I am more spiritual than when I am at my play. Running is my active meditation. I allow my spirit to lead and my body and emotions follow. Sometimes I pray when I run. It is a time when God and I have our best talks and shared time. For me, prayer is talking to God and meditation is listening to my Higher Being. So I talk about how grateful I am for my body, it's motion, strength, and wisdom. I listen for forgiveness for my human shortcomings and my everyday blunders. When I become "one with the road" my spirit and body are united and I find peace with the world— within. It is during this peace I can dream. And running gives me the strength in body, mind, and spirit to follow my dreams.

When I play at my canoeing and am living the awesome beauty of God's wilderness, I am sometimes overwhelmed with gratefulness. I experience an exuberant sensation of well-being which ends in a spontaneous explosion of joy and a shout at God "YOU DONE GOOD!!" I cling to and cherish these special, shared moments with God.

Judaism

The traditional toast on many Jewish occasions is "*l'chaim*—to life!*" Life and a commitment to participate in it completely is very much at the heart of Judaism. Virtues of hospitality and justice are ways of insuring the good life for others, and others—the community—are central to Jewish thought.

Along these lines we might ask ourselves: Am I hospitable to my body? Do I treat it with respect and provide it with all that it needs for comfort and life? Do I nurture it with food and water rather than deprive and punish it (because we "broke our diet"). Am I just to it—for the sake of others? A serious question. If I am abusive, then others are affected. Not attending to stress IS a contributing factor in heart disease, high blood pressure, asthma—the list is very long. Our ill health certainly affects us directly and those with whom we live and work and play.

MARVEL Recently, during a particularly stressful day when I was "dumping" all over my husband, who had listened for sometime but was becoming weary with the burden, he touched me gently and said, "I think you need a run." And he was right. It is one of my better methods of dealing effectively with stress (as well as a bit of dumping) and I needed to be reminded of it—for his sake and mine.

• • •

More indirectly, others are affected by the higher rates of health insurance. We don't think to be concerned about how our actions affect others is yet another form of "Jewish guilt," we think it is heightened consciousness.

There is an image in Jewish scriptures which seems particularly important in our discussion of women and active spirituality. The image is that of Lot's wife. Literally, an image: a statue made of salt. The message from God had been to "go." To move. Clearly to let go of one way of being and trust in God enough to move away into another land—another place. The command was given so that she and the whole community could live. If they stayed put, they would die. The only instruction was not to look back . . . this was to be a clean break and it called for courage. Lot's wife (she has no other name, no name of her own) began to move, but she did not go far. She kept looking back to her old home, her old way of being. There was no life for her there. Life was in moving and going into new territory. Her spiritual call had been to the active path and she chose not to follow it.

I can ask myself:
"Have I been looking back?"
— at a body of twenty years ago?
— at attitudes of a year ago?
— or attitudes of ten years ago? (do they still give me life?)
— at feelings of the past which hold me down today?

How do I deal with "looking back" and standing statue-like in one place? The techniques of goal setting described in chapter 3 could be helpful here.

There are chapters in Sacred Scripture which describe the contemplative spiritual path; they are familiar to us: "Be still and know that I am God." But often the active ones aren't thought of as prayers. But how often do the leaders of the people go up into the mountains to encounter a living God? It sounds pretty aerobic to us. It adds to the balance of how one can experience God. In quiet, still prayer; in moving, dynamic, struggling prayer. Remember Jacob wrestling with the angel of God—all night until his hip was out of joint? And what of the Exodus itself? Is this not about movement, walking, being a part of the community, being with God? Not staying put in Egypt. Is it not about freedom? Whether we are Jewish or not, we can take seriously a call to go forth to freedom. Our bodies are an integral part of this calling forth, this spiritual journey. How can I walk across the desert without it? Ask yourself if now might not be a time of personal exodus into a new spiritual land.

Non-Denominational Spirituality

In his very fine book, *Spiritual Wellness,* John Pilch speaks of various characteristics of those who are spiritually well or who are on a journey toward wellness. These people are ones who can risk, who are not afraid to explore diverse traditions and ways of becoming more spiritually alive and he says that one becomes more risky one step at a time. Do I dare try a Zen approach to my swimming? Cycling? Walking? Just for today? Dare I try a new group identity? *I am a runner. I am a swimmer. I am a racquetball player.* In taking the risk of a new identification,

I risk changing. I risk trying new things and being viewed in a different way by others—new friends, old friends, family. Risky business. My values may change. Our (perhaps hidden) child could be a spiritual guide for us when we want to risk, but have forgotten how. (see chapter 8)

Pilch also says that having identifiable values and striving to live by them is also a part of spiritual wellness. And how do I know what my values are? Ask yourself honestly:

How do I spend my time, my money, my life energy?
What and whom do I value?
Is it wholeness and balance, compassion, truthfulness, enlightenment?
What am I willing to do to obtain the things I value?
Could my body be part of my journey towards them?

These questions are spiritually important and yet they do not require a religious affiliation. Many times we hear women say, "Oh, I don't go to church; I guess I'm not very spiritual." It's a poor guess. Before there were churches and synagogues there were people who were spiritual. People who pondered the beginnings and ends of existence, who wondered about how to live, and how to live in relation to creation and other folks. It is very hard to find a woman who does not believe in something or some One. She may have a hard time naming it, she may be searching. But she is spiritually alive. This spirituality needs affirmation, not just denominational definition.

Then there is the matter of virtue, or good habits. Karl Menninger, a psychologist who knew the importance of spiritual wellness, asks the impertinent question in a book of the same title "What ever became of sin?" Perhaps it is also important to ask, "What ever became of virtue?" Is it irrelevant to living the good life?

"Virtue" comes from the Latin word *vir* which translates as "male." It translates as male, but it means strong, capable. Women are and can be strong and capable. We need strong and capable models to show us how to be virtuous. It is more effective than reading about women in a book to have someone live a life in such a way that the world is better. We are better for their having been on this planet. Right now this planet needs virtuous women and men. People who are patient, temperate, kind, merciful, generous; those who have shown fortitude and courage. What courage it takes to "Know Thyself" and LIVE thyself.

No, we don't think virtue is obsolete. We think it is a critical spiritual necessity if we are to "have life abundantly" to celebrate *l'chaim*, to survive.

Twelve-Step Spirituality

For over 50 years spiritual growth has been facilitated by various groups which focus on what are internationally referred to as twelve-step programs. These programs include Alcoholics Anonymous (AA), Al-Anon (for families and friends of substance abusers), Overeaters Anonymous (OA), Adult Children of Alcoholics (ACOA), and Co-Dependents Anonymous (CODA).

Twelve-step programs clearly are an important contemporary form of non-denominational spirituality. We think it is appropriate to briefly discuss at this point how twelve-step programs have been a catalyst for many women's spiritual awakening.

First, a bit of speculation. Why are so many people of such diverse cultures, ages, economic situations and religious backgrounds—and no religious backgrounds—helped by twelve-step programs? One reason seems apparent: during this century there have been enormous spiritual vacuums in people's lives which these programs fulfill. One of these vacuums is lack of support from others or a sense of real community.

For some, traditional religions have not provided the experience of belief which people need and seek. We emphasize the "experience" of belief because in theory or dogma most of the tenets of the twelve-step programs are contained in orthodox religious beliefs. Many memorize words of belief in God as a personal source of power, forgiveness and love but the words have been just that, words, not incorporated ways of living. Steps three, four, and nine, for example, do refer to experiencing this personal power, forgiveness, and love. The "fearless moral inventory" of step four is certainly related to Christian and Hebrew belief and practice. For some Christians and Jews it has not been experienced before in the same spiritually powerful way as for those who follow the paths of the twelve steps.

We would also note in this spiritual vacuum that addictions of various kinds (drugs, foods, cigarettes, shopping, other people) are often attempts by women to fill a need for Something or Someone. Into an empty or frustrating, angry, lonely, or powerless situation, these substances are falsely perceived as offering a temporary powerful, concrete satisfaction. The belief is that chocolate can be counted on to please, that an accumulation of goods will increase self-worth, that cigarettes do satisfy, and the other person will always be there. The person abusing the substance does not feel powerful; she does not feel that the holy or Higher Power in life is within her, but rather outside her grasp. She accepts it in various forms which she uses (abuses) and upon which she is dependent.

These addictions can also be false idols of worship. By this we mean that the person using them believes that they can bring life (the abundant *l'chaim* mentioned before) to the one depending on them. It is almost as if little shrines are set up in their honor. Their uses are often displayed and/or ritualized. Belief in their power to change one's life is focused outside, the interior life of the spirit is somehow lost or misplaced.

Addictions might also be viewed as spiritual dragons needing the taming approach rather than hatred and slaying. Only through understanding of one's needs and one's Higher Power can one effectively deal with dragons of addiction.

The twelve-step programs are programs which call the participant into reality, assessment, and primarily a new life and a new way of being and celebrating. Working the program means celebrating daily that precious gift for which one is mysteriously responsible and yet relating to One more powerful than self alone. This is a deeply spiritual reality and has shown itself of significant importance in millions of lives.

HOW TO GET SPIRITUAL ABOUT THE PHYSICAL

Gurus and sages admonish their novices to "learn to overcome obstacles to your spiritual goals." Different activities can provide different spiritual messages. For example, bicycle hill climbing or touring, cross-country running, walking, or skiing require one to overcome obstacles, both within yourself and outside of yourself. Sometimes in these sports you know when the obstacles are coming up, often you do not. One can learn how to deal with the unexpected and difficult while pursuing these physical activities. One can grow in spiritual insight through the activities themselves.

Almost all athletics teach endurance and proper use of power. The specific link between endurance exercises and spiritual pursuits is obvious in traditions like Kung Fu, Kajukimbo, and other martial arts which originally were spiritual paths and ways of being.

How about "go with the flow"? Good spiritual advice. You can learn much about it through scuba diving (no one can swim against dangerous currents for very long) or especially through canoeing. Have you been paddling up stream? Fighting and struggling against the water only slows one down, throws one off balance, off course and upsets the boat. It is far more difficult to struggle; it usurps the paddler's energy and absorbs one's senses. The beauty, the poetry of motion, the joy is gone.

"Enjoyable"—A much overlooked spiritual word.

CATHARINE I once heard a lecture by a Tibetan Buddhist lama who spoke eloquently and seriously about joy as a way to wisdom. "The way of suffering," he said, "is seen as the only way to become wise; this is not true. Do not forget the path of joy."

• • •

Joy changes us and enhances our life. The simple joy of our bodies can be a fine place to begin spiritual journeying. Pay attention to the joy of your body in motion, experience the joy of sweat and sun, and water; the joy of heart, lungs, muscles working well. "Be," as Emerson said, "a good animal" and know a little more about joy, about happiness.

CATHARINE One of the most spiritual spaces for me, more filled with awe and wonder than a cathedral, is in the sea. The vast waters prompt thoughts of *Genesis* and the beginnings of all cellular life in water. The beginning of my life in the waters of my mother's womb. Here in the deep, as I scuba dive into another dimension, it is easy for me to be in touch with the sacred and to know that I am sacred too. It is easy to be grateful for life and for creation. A creation that includes the creative minds which invented the aqua lung so that I am able to plunge into the depths. The psalmist David missed out on this, so I must sing my own songs of praise to God and the fishes.

• • •

If this chapter has sounded a bit like an "examination of conscious" or an inventory of self, perhaps it is. We don't apologize for something so spiritually old fashioned, or secularly modern. Religious traditions have had various forms of this activity for thousands of years.

What we've been talking about is, quite simply, the sacred. That which is holy. We have said that the holy is whole—it cannot ignore the body—and that the primary sacred space is one's body. Here (and really only through the body) one can encounter the living God. This encounter—this sacred time—may take place in one's mind, through one's feeling of God's presence, and/or through motion. Some women pursue the sacred almost exclusively through the mind. We are writing this book to invite women to consider a sacred journey which includes the wisdom of the body in motion.

Recommended Reading

Woman Spirit Rising: A Feminist Reader in Religion, ed. Carol P. Christ and Judith Plaskow. Harper Forum Books, New York, 1979.

Listening to Our Bodies, The Rebirth of Feminine Wisdom, Stephanie Demetrakopoulos. Beacon Press, Boston, 1983.

Wellness Spirituality, John Pilch. Crossroad, New York, 1985.

8

Motivating attrACTIVE Women for Life

*Why waste a perfectly good life just sitting around
wanting somebody to invite you to do something
when you could get busy, do it yourself, and
include some of your friends in it?*

Kay Morris Seidell

So . . . after a good beginning, how do I keep on being an
attrACTIVE woman? How do I make my sport or activity a real
part of my life, like brushing my teeth, or reading the news-
paper? Consider the following guidelines.

Be Active One Day at a Time

"For life"—"forever" is a long time. The very thought can
act as a barrier to my goal. Break "forever" into days since all
any of us have is today. Today is important, and taking care of
one day at a time is a very trite and very powerfully true ad-
monition. Our observation is that when one pays attention to
today, the todays have a way of building up into a life-style that
does include activity. However, each day does require a focus
upon being active. You do have to ask yourself the question,
"When will I go _____ today?" You have to think
about it. Only then will you be able to make a decision and act
upon it. On one, two, even three days of the week you may
decide NOT to be aerobically active. Sometime you may plan
a week off. That's fine. But do think about yourself as an active
person who is deciding to be inactive temporarily. Deciding not
to be aerobically active today is the exception; *being active is how
I usually live.*

Think of Myself as Active

So changing the way I think about myself is the first step in being motivated for life and focusing on now. How do I do this? I can take time to use my imagination; I see myself as I run or dance. I can get a clear picture of how this feels, smells and sounds. I can talk to myself—"I am an active person."—"I am becoming an athletic woman."

Hang Around with Active Women and Men

Other people are powerful motivators, so spend time with them. If you don't—if all your friends and associates are sedentary—your chances are slim that you will change your lifestyle.

MARVEL When I join my friends for early morning weekend runs it truly is rejuvenating. We talk, share, laugh. Once a friend suggested that he thought our jaws were getting a lot more exercise than our legs! He was probably right but so what, we have a great time. I remember running ahead of the group on a steep, long hill and my friend Mary Jo saying later "I love the feeling of power I experience when we women run together! We pull each other to the top like huge magnets. We are lifelines to each other." Indeed we are; there is a lot to be gained from hanging around active people.

• • •

We all need to get some understanding of and encouragement for our active life-styles. We need to hear that how we have chosen to live is valuable to another person. If all we hear is that we "must be crazy" to be riding or walking "in this kind of weather"—"at your age," then it's a lot harder to keep on believing in what we have found to be true. Very strong-willed women can do it—all power to them—but a lot of us get in that swim or run if we get recognition at some time from others who spend their time in the water or on the road.

Be on the Look-out for Mentors

MARVEL My mother has been an endless source of inspiration to me. She was out running several times a week long before it was a thing to do and was active in getting programs for others started too. Recently I was speaking at a health promotion conference for teachers and listened to a workshop on how to implement physical activity into the curriculum. A teacher from California was leading a group on how he built his social studies, geography, math, and health programs around his students running every day and adding up their mileage to run across America. I just smiled and said to myself, "Gosh, my Mom had her grade three kids in Coaldale, Alberta, running across Canada over twenty years ago!" It seems she has always been a little ahead of her time and there is always something to reach for.

CATHARINE I have really been inspired by other women— especially older women—who are active. It's not something they do on special occasions or for "show," they just take the time to "do their thing." And they keep on. Into their 50s, 60s, 70s, 90s . . . and I am so grateful to them. I don't think I could go on without their examples. Now I have the opportunity to do that same thing for younger women. When I go up to the starting line in a bicycle road race or time trial the young women look at me. (I don't look twenty—or thirty.) One said to me, "Hey, that's neat. When I see you here I think 'I can be doing this for a long, long time!'" Well, she might have left out one of the "longs," but I was glad that my presence had given her hope in her ability to continue to be an active woman.

• • •

When we read about 85-year-old Ruth Rothfarb running her seventh marathon we are so excited . . . for her and for ourselves. Ruth Rothfarb didn't start running until she was 72. She says, "I'm not remarkable." We want to respect that assessment instead of arguing with her, because to argue with her and make her out to be so unique gives us, and many other women, permission to be "ordinary" sedentary older women. Ruth goes on to say that she started to run for fun and found that it was something to do for herself that she couldn't buy. She doesn't compare herself to others; she runs for herself and when she can't run anymore (she notices that she is slowing down) then she says she'll walk. For Ruth running *is* a part of the way she is Ruth.

Try Competition

Ruth Rothfarb uses another motivator. Formal competition. Not just keeping track of her times when she's out, but she shows up on a certain day, at a certain time and she runs with others. NOTE: we said "she runs *with* others." Competition doesn't always mean running (walking, cycling, etc.) *against* others . . . or against others exclusively. It is because of the latter, narrow view, that many women avoid competition. Or vocally oppose it. Some feminists believe women ought not to compete . . . it's a "male" thing and very destructive.

We disagree. While we won't insist that all women "should" compete (we would not "should" on you for the world!), we do want to address the topic because competition can play a vital part in continuing motivation for being involved in sport or play.

First of all, to be competitive is not a male or female thing. It is part of human nature. It crosses cultures and forms of government. Russians want "better" running shoes; Americans want "better" burgers. Human beings *do compare* and it is not always a negative or destructive thing to do. When we go to a potluck we compare our salad, desert, etc., to others and in the process we often discover a different way of doing things. We change our old ways, and create a new way for ourselves that suits us better because we *did* compare—or compete. Women have been competing at state fairs for years. Those blue ribbons for quilts and canned peaches were not destructive of any other women. They were fun and satisfying and the events were pleasant social moments of sharing as well as comparing. Often they were opportunities to change for the better.

In New Mexico we have some of the finest runners in the country. They are Pueblo Indians who are usually considered non-competitive people by both culture and tradition. And they compete. All over the state, at Pike's Peak, in New York, all over the world. They see no conflict in values. Running is a way of life and competition has a way of bringing out the best in themselves. It gives pleasure to the tribe and others.

We have been impressed at how encouraging and helpful women are whom we meet at competitive events or while training for a particular event.

CATHARINE I want to share ways of bike handling on descents and turns; I want to learn how to hill climb better. It's when I am with other women, focused on a particular tour or race that these exchanges take place. I love my competitor, she brings out the best in me.

• • •

We are not saying that all competition is healthy and life-giving. Some is self-destructive and erodes relationships. But let's not throw the proverbial "baby out with the bath water." Ten-kilometer walks and runs can help us stay motivated and focused on being active. In and through these events we can meet other women who share similar values. They can also be ways of raising funds for causes such as heart and lung associations, multiple sclerosis, etc., or raising consciousness about important communal issues, like Take Back The Night, world peace, and hunger.

It seems to us when women refuse to be competitive or deny they are competitive that this denial manifests itself in other

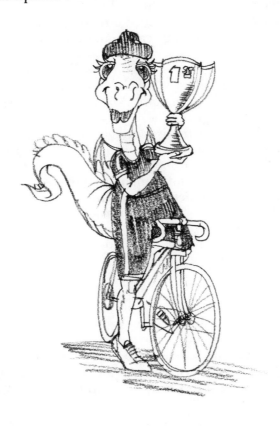

ways. One way is in comparing oneself to other women in how they look—what size and shape they are, what label is on their clothes, their hairstyle, or who they are seen with. The problem is that often these same women struggle with insecurities and have low self-esteem, so no matter what the comparison is they always come out on the bottom (which doesn't do a thing for their self-worth). We see this phenomenon repeatedly in women's support and therapy groups. Being competitive is natural and very human and the choice to be competitive with your activity seems much healthier than for the competitive nature to fester as underlying comparisons.

And very importantly, competition can be fun! That particular kind of fun that maybe we never had as little girls without a chance (because of sex or physique) to "go for the gold." A friend of ours was being challenged about his competitive skiing interest at his "late age" of 45 and his response shows how in touch he was with the child inside. "Remember," he said, "those little trophies they had in the eighth grade? They still have them." Sure, they don't measure our worth as human beings, but they can be fun and they can remind us that we are serious about our bodies.

Another thing which competition can teach us is that we can't always win. We can't always "do our best." This is an important thing to know in life in general. We are not failures if we fail or fall short of our goals. There are other days, other times to "go for it." We may surprise ourselves and others. Through competition we can learn how to be prepared for successes and/ or failure. We can learn how to move toward a goal—how to "peak" for an event and not demand of ourselves that we "peak" at all times. Many women burn themselves out because they demand of themselves a peak performance daily: at home, office, with friends and family. This is unrealistic. We think competition has the potential of "reality orientation" which is pretty important for today's women.

Be Realistic

Being in touch with reality is important for self-motivation in regards to the continuation of an active lifestyle. It is unrealistic to expect that 100 percent of the time I will be fully energized by my activity and enjoy it completely. If I demand that kind of satisfaction I am setting myself up for disappointment—and an excuse *not* to be active. But we can honestly say that about 85 to 90 percent of the time the pleasurable, refreshing, energizing aspects *are* there and they are worth the price of the 10 percent when they aren't. If the pleasure is gone most of the time, switch activities, or combine them. Don't use "burn-out" as an excuse to take to the couch.

Talk to Yourself

Motivation can be enhanced with self-talk. NOT put down talk! No "lazy-bum," "fat slob" put-downs, please. Treat yourself kindly. Encourage yourself. Remind yourself of your real goals (that 5K walk rather than this imminent "flop down"). Remind yourself that you are an active woman who wants to resemble that *today*. If you do choose not to go out, that's OK. Congratulate yourself on your good judgement. There is always tomorrow. If there are two or three "tomorrows" in a row, sit down and ask yourself if this is what you really want. If not, how and when will you return to an active life? We think you'd be understanding and supportive of your friends if they hit a snag in what they wanted out of life. Be as gentle with yourself. You deserve understanding and encouragement too.

Here is some self-talk to try out:

* Doing something (a little bit) is better than nothing.
* When I am active, I am attractive. I glow and glisten.
* I am dependable because I am not sick and depressed so frequently.
* I feel *alive, available, energized, capable, strong.*

Talk to Your Body

We are continually giving messages to our body. More often than not women are giving their bodies put-downs. What are you saying to yourself when you look in the mirror? Is it a continual rundown of "what a fat stomach" (chin, arms, etc.) or "my thighs are so ugly and flabby," or "I hate my rear end." When was the last time you thanked your thighs for carrying you around? Gave a bit of encouragement to your hair, or legs? It's a wonder the parts don't go out on strike. Do you have an old habit of bad mouthing your body? Begin to change the habit by trying positive talk for a week or so; give your body a break, and a boost.

Reward Your Body

Many of us remember receiving awards for excellence as little girls. We got gold stars, ribbons, pins, certificates, and prizes of all sorts. There was a great sense of satisfaction and pleasure in seeing tangible evidence of our achievements. Local clubs, merchants, cities, states, and provinces offer a great variety of events with awards for participants of differing abilities and ages. In both Canada and the USA there are national fitness awards with rather stiff, yet achievable criteria which afford that special opportunity of recognition. For further information on the requirements for awards in numerous fitness categories and sporting events contact your community sports and recreation centers, they will have local and national information. These "pats on the back" keep us motivated to move and move on.

Try Celebrating With Your Body

Celebrations are a lovely way to enhance our motivation and keep us going on with our goal of an active life-style. They offer a time of joy, of recognition, and possible reflection. Celebrations come in all sorts of packages. We celebrate anniversaries, beginnings and endings, changes, successes. We do this with cards, special meals, entertainments. Different cultures celebrate differently, some mark occasions with music, poetry, small gifts. Picking an activity as a way of celebrating can be very rewarding.

MARVEL My most memorable birthday was my 25th. I kayaked the Sjoa River in Norway to celebrate it and to celebrate me. Later I learned from Torkle, our Norwegian guide, that I was probably the first woman to ever make the run. It is a celebration to treasure.

CATHARINE My husband and I celebrated our 50th birthdays by bicycling from Canada to Mexico. It was a glorious way to say to each other, "I'm glad you were born." It was a memorable way to reflect on a half century of living. We had a lot of fun planning it together and importantly it kept me motivated to ride regularly so that I had no difficulty with the terrain or long miles.

• • •

A changed image of self, inspiration of others, competition, self-understanding, self-talk, celebrating, these are some of your primary ways of keeping motivated TODAY. Secondarily, you might consider a few rewards such as those mentioned in chapter 3, especially the reward of equipment . . . or just consider a bit of new sporting equipment, period. It can give you a boost. A new pair of running shoes, a new aerobic dance outfit can boost your spirit and your performance. Along with a change in equipment can be a change in activity. Running year-round may lead to burn-out; if so, try some swimming, tap-dancing, hiking, or rope jumping as alternative aerobic activities. Some sports go quite well in combination. For example, ice skating in the winter and cycling in the warmer months. Or cross-country skiing, one of the best aerobic activities of all, combined with walking, running or cycling during "off season." You may be able to think of all sorts of combinations which can keep you looking forward to playful activity which gives you a sense of well-being and is also fun.

CATHARINE I don't know whether I cycle so that I can cross-country ski and scuba dive or the other way around. All are very enjoyable and very different experiences, physically and spiritually. I do know that doing one activity helps keep me prepared and motivated for the other. I'm just the kind of person who would get tired of just one sport—I'd run the risk of becoming inactive if I were developing only one form of play.

• • •

Yes, there is some effort required in staying motivated. *You* are the only one that can motivate yourself—no one can do it for you, and *you can't motivate anyone else.* You are the one who decides to be inspired by other active women. The longer you are active, the less effort it takes to stay motivated. Being active becomes a habit—a good habit—a virtue. Automatically, you will think of being active; automatically, you will plan your week including your business trip or vacation, around your activity. You will travel with walking shoes and sweat pants or swim suit. It takes time to develop this good habit. But it took time, per-haps years, to *not* play. When we were in grade school, we automatically played. It *was* part of our daily life.

It can be again. There is a child that still lives inside each one of us. For some it has been years since that child has had a chance to really be alive. Some women have become masters at taking life so seriously and being *perfect* that the child is pushed way out of sight. Possibly they grew up too fast, had the responsibilities of an adult too soon. Maybe they had an alcoholic parent or a very nonfunctional family and never learned to play even as a youngster. Whatever the reason, the child is still there, somewhere, and we bet she is aching to get out and stretch a little. Learning to play as an adult is not easy. It takes some time to practice and to not feel "silly" or "embarrassed." Women in our groups share some of their play experiences with us like singing while they drive, dressing for Halloween, dancing in the living room, and laughing out loud when reading a funny story.

There is so much we can learn from our child if we would trust her and listen. Some lessons she might be trying to teach us are: "Life is too short to get hung up on some of the details of living such as dishes and dust."

MARVEL Sometime in the past year, I was flying home from a meeting with my husband when we got in this "heavy" discussion about life's goals, etc. and it led from one philosophical thing to another. All of a sudden I turned to him and said "You know, Jeffrey, sometimes I get really confused with myself. I feel like the real Marvel is this little kid running around inside a grown-up body, doing grown-up things like giving talks, attending meetings, making decisions, having philosophical discussions but the real me is this little kid having a great time messing around, giggling, playing, and not being serious at all. I wonder which one of me other people see?" He laughed softly and said "Marvel, your little kid is oozing out all the time. Why do you think I married you?" We both thoroughly enjoy our child within and our child has so much to offer us. I told him later that the thing in life I wanted to be remembered for was living and sharing my concept of "the playful child is mother to the woman." It has been so very powerful for me.

• • •

Play is an option for our daily lives. The child inside each one of us *can* be the mother to the attrACTIVE woman we are becoming. Perhaps this child is our most powerful motivation. Give her a chance to teach us the wisdom born in our bodies.

Recommended Reading

Runner's World, Bicycling Magazine, Walking, Shape, Women's Sports and Fitness Magazine, or any one which catches your eye and reinforces your active habit.

APPENDIX A

FITNESS SCALES

AEROBIC PROGRAMS

Walking
Running
Cycling
Swimming

STATIONARY PROGRAMS

Cycling
Running
Rope Skipping
Winter Sports

COOPER FITNESS SCALES
12 Minute Walking/Running Test
Distance (Miles) Covered in 12 Minutes

FITNESS CATEGORY	AGES (YEARS)				
	20-29	30-39	40-49	50-59	60+
Very Poor	<.96	<.94	<.88	<.84	<.78
Poor	.96-1.11	.95-1.05	.88-.98	.84-.93	.78-.86
Fair	1.12-1.22	1.06-1.18	.99-1.11	.94-1.05	.87-.98
Good	1.23-1.34	1.19-1.29	1.12-1.24	1.06-1.18	.99-1.09
Excel.	1.35-1.45	1.30-1.39	1.25-1.34	1.19-1.30	1.10-1.18
Super.	>1.46	>1.40	>1.35	>1.31	>1.19

< means "less than"; > means "more than"

1.5 Mile Run Test
Time (Minutes)

FITNESS CATEGORY	AGES				
	20-29	30-39	40-49	50-59	60+
Very Poor	>19:01	>19:31	>20:01	>20:31	>21:01
Poor	18:-19:00	19:-19:30	19:30-20:	20:-20:30	21:-21:31
Fair	15:5-18:3	16:3-19:0	17:3-19:3	19:-20:0	19:3-20:3
Good	13:3-15:5	14:3-16:3	15:5-17:3	16:3-19:0	17:3-19:3
Excel.	12:3-13:3	13:0-14:3	13:5-15:5	14:3-16:3	16:3-17:3
Superior	<12:30	<13:00	<13:45	<14:30	<16:30

12-Minute Swimming Test
Distance (Yards) Swum in 12 Minutes

FITNESS CATEGORY	20-29	30-39	40-49	50-59	60+
Very Poor	<300	<250	<200	<150	<150
Poor	300-399	250-349	200-299	150-249	150-199
Fair	400-499	350-449	300-399	250-349	200-299
Good	500-599	450-549	400-499	350-449	300-399
Excellent	>600	>550	>500	>450	>400

12 Minute Cycling Test
(Cooper bases this on 3-Speed or less, we would use it for any bicycle)
Distance (Miles) Cycled in 12 Minutes

FITNESS CATEGORY	20-29	30-39	40-49	50-59	60+
Very Poor	<1.5	<1.25	<1.0	<.75	<.75
Poor	1.5-2.49	1.25-2.24	1.0-1.99	.75-1.49	.75-1.24
Fair	2.5-3.5	2.25-3.24	2.0-2.99	1.50-2.5	1.25-2.0
Good	3.5-4.5	3.25-4.24	3.0-3.99	2.5-3.5	2.0-2.99
Excellent	>4.5	>4.25	>4.0	>3.5	>3.0

The above fitness "tests" are from *The Aerobics Program for Total Well-Being* by Dr. Kenneth H. Cooper, Bantam Books/M. Evans & Co. Inc., New York, 1982.

We include them for your convenience. We urge you to begin a fitness program *wherever* you are and feel free to define your own progress. *Trust your body first* and any chart second. The important thing is to begin to move, and continue to do so— not where you fit into someone else's test or chart but where you are comfortable and where your activity level is or will be aerobic. We think Dr. Cooper would agree with us.

AEROBIC PROGRAMS

Walking Program

Note: These programs are *guidelines*. Listen to your body—especially your heart rate—to determine if this progression is right for you. Check in chapter 2 for your maximum heart rate and work at 60 to 75 percent of that. It may take 12 weeks or more to work through this walking program. If one week's goal is not met, REPEAT THE WEEK. There is no rush. Enjoy the activity, and enjoy the benefits.

This program is based on walking 3 to 5 times each week.

WEEKS	STRETCH & WARM UP	TARGET ZONE	STRETCH & COOL DOWN	TOTALS
1	5 min.	Walk briskly 5 min.	5 min.	15 min.
2	5 min.	Walk briskly 7 min.	5 min.	17 min.
3	5 min.	Walk briskly 9 min.	5 min.	19 min.
4	5 min.	Walk briskly 11 min.	5 min.	21 min.
5	5 min.	Walk briskly 13 min.	5 min.	23 min.
6	5 min.	Walk briskly 15 min.	5 min.	25 min.
7	5 min.	Walk briskly 18 min.	5 min.	28 min.
8	5 min.	Walk briskly 20 min.	5 min.	30 min.
9	5 min.	Walk briskly 23 min.	5 min.	33 min.
10	5 min.	Walk briskly 26 min.	5 min.	36 min.
11	5 min.	Walk briskly 28 min.	5 min.	38 min.
12	5 min.	Walk briskly 30 min.	5 min.	40 min.

Walking Notes:

Equipment The nice thing about walking is that it is convenient and requires only a minimum of equipment, i.e., proper shoes. Only recently have there been specific sport walking shoes (there are articles about them which you may want to read). Basically, use comfortable shoes with plenty of room for your toes. Good socks make a difference. Try different socks and be sure to change them often.

Clothing Anything comfortable and loose. In cold weather protect your hands and head. Remember sunglasses and sunscreen when necessary.

Tips Hold your body erect, straight, and shoulders back. Instead of letting your arms hang down, keep your elbows bent (this way your hands won't swell as much), and allow for a gentle forward swinging motion across your front (not side to side). Your arms set the pace as you move them. Keep your hands relaxed, not in a tight fist. Take comfortable length strides— they don't have to be long. If you walk with a friend whose pace is slower than yours, wear a back pack with a book or two in it so your heart rate will increase. This allows the two of you to walk together and both meet your Target Heart Rate Zone. Keep your toenails trimmed.

RUN/WALK PROGRAM

For stretching illustrations and heart rate charts see chapter 2.

WEEKS	STRETCH & WARM UP	TARGET ZONE	STRETCH & COOL DOWN	TOTALS
1	5 min.	walk briskly 10 min.	walk slowly 3 min. stretch 2 min.	20 min.
2	5 min.	walk 5 min. run 1 min. 2x	walk slowly 3 min. stretch 2 min.	22 min.
3	5 min.	walk 5 min. run 3 min. 2x	walk slowly 3 min. stretch 2 min.	26 min.
4	5 min.	walk 4 min. run 5 min. 2x	walk slowly 3 min. stretch 2 min.	28 min.
5	5 min.	walk 4 min. run 5 min. 2x	walk slowly 3 min. stretch 2 min.	28 min.
6	5 min.	walk 4 min. run 6 min. 2x	walk slowly 3 min. stretch 2 min.	30 min.
7	5 min.	walk 4 min. run 7 min. 2x	walk slowly 3 min. stretch 2 min.	32 min.
8	5 min.	walk 4 min. run 8 min. 2x	walk slowly 3 min. stretch 2 min.	34 min.

(cont.)

WEEKS	STRETCH & WARM UP	TARGET ZONE	STRETCH & COOL DOWN	TOTALS
9	5 min.	walk 4 min. run 9 min. 2x	walk slowly 3 min. stretch 2 min.	36 min.
10	5 min.	walk 4 min. run 13 min.	walk slowly 3 min. stretch 2 min.	27 min.
11	5 min.	walk 4 min. run 15 min.	walk slowly 3 min. stretch 2 min.	29 min.
12	5 min.	walk 4 min. run 17 min.	walk slowly 3 min. stretch 2 min.	31 min.
13	5 min.	walk 2 min. run slowly 2 run 17 min.	walk slowly 3 min. stretch 2 min.	31 min.
14	5 min.	walk 1 min. run slowly 3 run 17 min.	walk slowly 3 min. stretch 2 min.	31 min.
15	5 min.	run slowly 3 run 17 min.	walk slowly 3 min. stretch 2 min.	30 min.

Running and Walking Notes

Equipment Shoes are the main thing. Getting good ones is important; a proper fit is essential. Take a well-worn pair of shoes with you when you shop for new ones. They will indicate your wear patterns and be good information on the style of your stride and whether you pronate (wear inward) or supenate (wear outward). There are shoes available to help correct either situation. Try shoes on with the type of sock you plan to wear. Walk and run around in them on a hard surface (not just the carpet of the store). A "good" store encourages this. Take your time—try on many styles. Be sure the heel area is narrow enough that you don't slip or you may have blister problems. A sturdy bottom sole increases the wear of the shoe. Replace shoes as necessary—keeping your shoes just for running will extend their life! Expect to buy shoes slightly larger than dress shoe sizes, and plan to spend $40 to $60 (1989 prices).

140

Socks need to fit comfortably—any folds or wrinkles result in blisters.

A support/sport bra is a must, (see page 149.)

Clothing Wear a hat, sunscreen, sunglasses, or sweat band when necessary. Use loose fitting clothing and be sure shorts have a comfortable liner with no rough seams to irritate. Wear layers in cool or cold weather. A good combination is lightweight "polypropylene" long underwear with loose fitting running pants and jacket on top. For rainy weather a "Gortex" suit is very comfortable since it keeps the wet out and can still "breath." Keep your hands and head covered. Dry out your shoes immediately, not over direct heat—most shoes have an inner sole that easily pulls out. Wear reflective clothing (vest) when running on the road.

Tips Run with your body erect and straight. Hold your arms bent at the elbow with your hands relaxed, not clenched in a tight fist. Try not to rotate your upper body from the waist with shoulders going back and forth. Very little upper body motion is necessary. Don't make drastic changes in *how* you run. Don't try to run on your toes or the ball of your foot if you normally do not. As with normal walking most people's heel will touch first. Think about a fluid motion and your body moving smoothly, not in a pounding, jarring fashion. Some women find rubbing some Vaseline on their inner thighs prevents rubbing and irritation. Keep your toenails trimmed. A good running surface is level, smooth, and has a little cushion. An even, non-paved road or trail is ideal. Grass is easy to trip on. Be sure the surface is level—a sloped beach or road can aggravate your knees. Staying out of traffic is optimum. Be aware of your personal safety, *be street smart.* Running with company is a good idea. Have identification on your person at all times and a quarter for an emergency phone call. Building a slow, solid base is important. Most injuries occur when *too much, too soon, too fast, too hard* is tried. Your aim is to be active for life, not to run a certain number of miles. Be patient; talk to other women about how they got started and have kept up their programs.

Swimming Program

This program is based on 3 to 4 times per week. Attention to maximum heart rate is important. It is often recommended to stay in the Starting Target Heart Rate Zone of 65 to 70 percent of MHR. See chapter 2.

If swimming 10 minutes is too difficult for starters, then swim what you can and spend the rest of the time holding on to the side and kicking or using a kick board. Just keep moving for the 10 minutes. Many prefer to use a variety of strokes when they "do their time"; this is fine as long as the heart rate is in the target zone.

Most swimmers would agree that a crawl/freestyle is more difficult, a side stroke more restful. Alternate strokes, then increase the amount of "crawl time" as you progress.

Remember: Time spent swimming and heart rate are more important items to note than distance. We use distance for convenience. Remember, also, that it is better to stay at one level and complete it for a whole week, before advancing.

WEEK	WARM-UP IN WATER	DISTANCE (YARDS)	TIME	STRETCH
1	5 min.	200	15 min.	3 min.
2	5 min.	250	15 min.	3 min.
3	5 min.	300	12 min.	3 min.
4	5 min.	300	10 min.	3 min.
5	5 min.	400	13 min.	3 min.
6	5 min.	400	12 min.	3 min.
7	5 min.	500	14 min.	3 min.
8	5 min.	500	13 min.	3 min.
9	5 min.	600	16 min.	3 min.
10	5 min.	700	19 min.	3 min.
11	5 min.	800	22 min.	3 min.
12	5 min.	900	23 min.	3 min.

Swimming Notes

Equipment Swimsuit and goggles are the bare necessities. The swimsuit should not be a fashion one, cut out here and there and everywhere! Get a swimsuit in a sporting goods shop and note the high cut neck. This is to prevent a lot of drag from water which will slow you down. Nylon and lycra are the primary materials for suits. Chlorine is hard on them; they fade and wear out rather quickly. Goggles must fit properly so they need to be tried on in the store and then adjusted in the water. After several attempts you will get a good seal and then not have to be concerned.

Equipment options include hand paddles, kick boards, and styrafoam to put between your legs. These accessories allow you to concentrate on one aspect of swimming at a time (e.g., working on arm strokes, or leg kicks) and also can add variety to a swim session. One friend does two laps of leg work (holding on to a board) and then two lengths not using her legs at all, just working on her arms.

For those prone to sinus infections, nose plugs are a must. Ear plugs are important for others. Although not allowed in competition, many women who have trouble mastering smooth breathing use a snorkle. If this helps you enjoy the sport more, use it and get the aerobic benefit of swimming. Swim caps are not a necessary piece of equipment unless your hair is long, then caps are required. Some women with short hair choose to use caps in order to swim faster or more smoothly; caps do not keep your hair dry!

Tips Hair and skin are concerns which keep some women away from swimming. Usually, swimmers choose short hairstyles, but not all. Braids are the solution of many. Whether long or short, hair frequently in chlorinated water needs special attention or it will discolor and/or begin to "feel funny". There are several brands of shampoo made especially for swimmers and we recommend using them and similarly prepared conditioners. Most importantly, be sure you wet your hair thoroughly before entering the pool; in this way your hair can't absorb so much of the chlorine.

Skin will get dry after repeated swim sessions so using lotions, creams or oils will help. *But do not use the oils and lotions before going into the pool.* This is not looked upon favorably by pool owners and managers.

Pool etiquette: When the "lap lanes" are crowded (more than two persons in a lane) then "circle swim" is in order. This means that you swim in the RIGHT SIDE of the lane, turn and return in the RIGHT SIDE of the lane.

Many pools have Red Cross safety checks. When this happens a loud horn blows and all must clear the pool until further notice from the lifeguard.

Bicycling Program

This program is based on 3 to 5 times per week. Because a lot of us do not live in completely flat areas, there will be differences in time spent for distance covered. These are guidelines, or approximations. What you are working towards is sustained activity for 25 to 30 minutes. Stretching is recommended before and after cycling as well as the "warm-up time" indicated.

WEEK	WARM-UP	DISTANCE	SPIN	TIME
1	5 min.	4-4.5 mi.	65 rpm	20:00
2	5 min.	4-4.5 mi.	70 rpm	18:00
3	5 min.	5-5.5 mi.	70 rpm	24:00
4	5 min.	5-5.5 mi.	75 rpm	22:00
5	5 min.	5-5.5 mi.	75 rpm	20:00
6	5 min.	6-6.5 mi.	80 rpm	26:00
7	5 min.	6-6.5 mi.	80 rpm	24:00
8	5 min.	7-7.5 mi.	80 rpm	30:00
9	5 min.	7-7.5 mi.	80 rpm	28:00
10	5 min.	7-8.0 mi.	80 rpm	30:00

Note: RPM (revolutions per minute) is given to emphasize the importance of "spinning," e.g., not pushing a tough, high gear. This is a tendency for many who want to get a "good" workout . . . NOT TRUE. Spinning with LESS tension is better for your body and gives you an excellent workout. (The top competitive athletes spin 95-100+). It sounds technical, but is important and easy to determine if you have a digital watch or a second hand on a watch. Just count how many times you pedal a complete circle in 60 seconds . . . that's your rpm.

Cycling Notes

Equipment What kind of bicycle to buy is a lot more involved decision than what kind of swimsuit to buy! And a lot more expensive.

Your taste in bicycling will determine whether you go for a mountain bike, touring bike, or racing bike. Quality and fit are the most important aspects of any type of bicycle. Do not buy a "ladies bike" from a general merchandise store. They are heavy, of uneven quality, and have no mechanic to back them up, or help you out as you get to know your machine. A qualified bicycle shop will have sales people who can help you get equipment which will meet your taste and needs and which will fit. Be sure you are fitted by more criteria than standing over the frame. Check the seat height, and the length of the seat to handle bars.

Try the bike out (more than around the block) and talk to experienced riders about their bikes before you make a decision. There is good information available about bicycles; check out the special insert in *Women's Sports and Fitness Magazine* (February 1987) on women and bicycling equipment. *Bicycling Magazine,* June 1987, and Feb., 1989, has a very good review of women's bikes.

Be sure your bicycle is equipped with water bottles, frame pump, and patch kit (yes, there ARE flats and you need to learn how to change them).

There are lots of other items that can be added to your basic bike, but these are the essentials.

Clothing Helmet (a MUST), gloves, shorts (those stretchy "ugly black ones" are *much* more comfortable), and eye protection. In changeable weather, or on cool days, using layers of clothing is a good idea.

Tips Spinning has already been mentioned. Having a friend who rides and can help you learn a few tricks of the trade would be a great asset. If you're on your own, be sure to "get out of the saddle" (off the seat) every 20 minutes or so. Drink lots of water (BEFORE you are thirsty), about one water bottle an hour, and eat if you are on a ride over 60 minutes.

Automobile traffic is a problem, no doubt about it. Know your traffic rights (you ARE allowed to travel in the right lane— not the gutter!), obey traffic signals, make eye contact with drivers, and watch out for side mirrors on parked trucks, drivers opening doors, cars behind you passing and turning left in front of you. Drivers often don't realize that bikes are going fast or that most of us are strapped into the pedals with toe clips or other systems which make it a bit harder to stop suddenly.

Stationary Cycling Program

WEEK	SPIN RPM	TIME	HR AFTER EXERCISE	FREQUENCY X PER WEEK
1	55	6:00	17-22	3
2	55	8:00	17-22	3
3	55	10:00	17-22	3
4	60	12:00	18-23	4
5	60	14:00	18-23	4
6	65	16:00	18-24	4
7	65	18:00	18-24	3-5
8	65	20:00	18-24	3-5
9	70	20:00	18-24	3-5
10	75	20:00	18-24	3-5
11	75	22:00	18-24	4-5
12	80	22:00	18-24	4-5
13	85	23:00	18-24	4-5
14	85	25:00	18-24	4-5

Stationary Program Notes

Warm up by stretching first and going slowly for 3 min. before "getting up to speed." Cool down the same way. The charts are an approximation—when in doubt, *check your heart rate for your age.* Keep a glass of water handy to sip, wear a sweat band. Some women use an electric fan blowing on them because they get hot. Many listen to music, T.V. or tapes . . . stationary cycling can get boring so think ahead about how to eliminate this barrier.

Stationary Running, Rope Skipping, Stair Climbing

Like stationary cycling these programs call for:

1) warm up (3 to 5 minutes)
2) beginning with 7 to 8 minutes of aerobic level effort
3) increasing GRADUALLY over a 10- to 14-week period to the following:
   running—15 min.
   rope skipping—15 min.
   stair climbing—13 min.

These activities are generally used to prepare for other sports, to allow for fitness training during periods of poor weather, or to build strength in a specific part of your body. They are handy for travel/vacation times because they don't require a lot of time or equipment. Headphones can be a great help in these activities, also.

Winter Sports

The most aerobic winter sports are:

• cross-country skiing (x-country)
• snow shoeing
• ice skating (continuously)

Downhill skiing generally isn't aerobic. *How* you do it, and how *long* you do it, is the key. The same is true with ice hockey. Both sports have lots of stops and starts, which means they aren't aerobic . . . may be fun though!

Winter sports can add variety to your attrACTIVE WOMAN program and, if you live in an area with dependable ice or snow, they can be your main focus in the winter.

The same rules apply: dress properly (layers)
                        warm up and cool down
                        keep track of your Heart Rate
                        progress gradually

AND ENJOY YOURSELF

APPENDIX B

FITNESS EXTRAS

Sports bras
Sunscreens
Sunglasses
Insect Repellant

SPORTS BRAS

Sports bras are a necessary consideration for being a comfortable attrACTIVE WOMAN. Whatever your particular needs, selecting a sports bra is important. Until recently it has been difficult for large breasted women to find sports bras in their sizes. This is no longer true. You may have to check with several shops, but it is worth the search.

The following are recommendations by our friend LaJean Lawson from *The Physician and Sports Medicine,* Vol. 15, No. 5, May 1987.

Which sports bra provides the best defense against motion-related breast discomfort and potential injury? The answer to this question depends on several variables, on which we base the following recommendations:

Cup Size. Large breasted women, who generally require more support to control motion, should select a more rigidly constructed bra than small-breasted women, who may find a stretchy bra adequately supportive and more comfortable.

Sport of Choice. Different sports often require varying amounts of arm involvement and range of motion. For sports requiring significant amount of overhead reaching, bra straps must stretch so as to prevent riding up of the bra over the breast. Sports requiring leg action and jogging without significant overhead reaching are well served by a bra with firm, nonstretch straps connected directly or almost directly to a non-elastic cup.

Fabric Preferences and Sensitivities. Sports bras are made in a wide variety of fibers, fabric weights, and firmness of construction. Choice should depend on intensity of activity, support needs, sensitivity to fiber, and climatic and seasonal conditions.

Protection Needs. A breast protector (a pad that can be inserted into the bra cup) may be desirable for women who participate in contact sports.

Quality of Design and Construction. Active women should look for a bra that has no irritating seams or fasteners next to the skin, nonslip straps, silhouettes that hold the breasts in a rounded shape close to the body, and firm, durable construction.

SUNSCREENS

Use sunscreen whenever you are out of doors—summer or winter. Purchase a brand containing both PABA (para-aminobenzoic acid) and benzone compounds (such as benzophenone or oxybenzone). You will then be protected against both UVA and UVB rays. Choose one with a Sun Protection Factor (SPF) of at least 15 and waterproof if you plan to play and get wet. Apply it ahead of time and reapply it frequently. For your sensitive and tender parts (ears, lips, nose) you can use an opaque sun block such as titanium dioxide or zinc oxide. Remember that harmful rays can burn even through a cloud cover. Some people may experience an adverse reaction to sunscreen products and need to consult a dermatologist.

SUNGLASSES

There are several things to look for in a pair of sunglasses. Be sure they block UV light. Labels that claim blockage of "100% UV" may be misleading. The only industry standards for UV absorption are those with "Z-80.3" printed on the frame. If you spend a lot of time out of doors you will need lenses which block blue light also. Be sure the lenses:

- are large enough (you might try a wraparound style)
- block enough visible light (you can't see your eyes)
- fit so they don't slip on your nose

If you spend hours driving or out of doors at a sport like cycling or skiing you may need lenses which are polarized, mirrored, gradient, or photochromic.

INSECT REPELLANT

There is a relatively safe, effective insect repellant called N, N-diethyltoluamide, known as DET or deet. Some of the chemical does enter the blood stream and for some women may cause an allergic reaction. The lower concentrations are safer but have to be applied more frequently. Don't use on broken skin or over cuts and scratches. When possible, instead of using repellants, cover up with clothing and tuck your pants into your socks.

Some Cautions: You are entering into a whole new world; there are a million gadgets, thing-am-a-bobs, and gimmicks. Some could be an asset to your enjoyment of a sport, others could merely cost you money, some are downright dangerous. Proceed with a good dose of common sense. Generally avoid anything that comes close to self-medicating—this would include using braces, or wraps. Physical problems and/or injuries need to be looked at by professionals.

APPENDIX C

TEN COMMANDMENTS FOR attrACTIVE WOMEN

Adapted from Runner's World, August 1987

1. *Increase your mileage and intensity gradually.* Only carefully integrate speed work into your schedule. Be aware of signs of overtraining (tired legs, insomnia, loss of appetite, increase in morning resting heart rate).
2. *Never run through an injury or illness.* If it hurts to run, don't. Swim or cycle until the injury heals. If you're sick, ease up. Listen to your body.
3. *Recover fully after races.* Avoid the urge to compete every weekend.
4. *Listen to your body.* If you feel tired or sluggish, fight the habit of muddling through a mediocre workout. Instead of suffering and risking injury, go easy or rest until you've regained your pep. Overtraining does more damage than undertraining.
5. *Incorporate regular easy days into your schedule.* Regardless of what anyone says. Easy workouts give your body time to recover and grow stronger.
6. *Always warm up.* Before any swim, ride, or run, and especially before competition. Your body performs best when given time to prepare for exercise. It's your best prevention for injuries.
7. *Always cool down.* Quitting abruptly not only shocks your system, but you'll pay for it the next day when the accumulated lactic acid saps your energy.
8. *Use proper equipment.* Check it regularly, and keep it in good repair.
9. *Drink and eat enough to fuel your muscles.* Drink 8 to 10 glasses of fluid per day and two cups for every hour of aerobic activity.
10. *Find a balance in your activities.* There is a danger in becoming too focused on sport; there are other joys and satisfactions which need to be experienced if one is to become a whole person. All the aerobic activity and training in the world is meaningless without the support of family, friends, and co-workers.

APPENDIX D

NUTRITION NOTES

Calcium
Iron
Vitamin C
Snacks

CALCIUM

FOOD SOURCES OF CALCIUM

FOOD	SERVING SIZE	CALCIUM* (MILLIGRAMS)	CALORIES*
Skim milk	8 oz.	290	90
Low-fat milk (2%)	8 oz.	290	120
Whole milk	8 oz.	290	160
Buttermilk	8 oz.	290	90
Yogurt (low-fat, plain)	8 oz.	250	110
Yogurt (low-fat, fruit-flavored)	8 oz.	250	260
Cheddar cheese	1 oz.**	210	110
Swiss cheese	1 oz.**	260	100
Cottage cheese (low-fat)	1 cup	150	120
Sardines with bones	3 oz.	300	225
Salmon with bones	3 oz.	250	180
Tofu (soybean curd)	4 oz.	150	80
Broccoli	1 cup	140	40

*Approximate values
**1 oz. of hard cheese is about equal to a 1½″ to 2″ cube
Note: 150 mg. calcium available from ½ cup of dark green vegetables except spinach, chard, and beet greens

There are many choices when it comes to getting calcium in your diet—sometimes women get really wrapped up in counting milligrams in this and that, and it becomes a lot of work. You really can get your day's supply of calcium from 20 cups of Brussels sprouts or 11 cups whipping cream! It might be easier to incorporate a few easy tips.

To Increase Calcium

- In salads use the dark green leaves (also high in vitamins A, B, D, E, and other minerals).
- Substitute grated cheese for butter on vegetables or bread—Parmesan is yummy!
- Garnish salads and soups with tofu.
- Add a ¼ cup of nonfat dry milk to recipes when you bake or make casseroles. Try it as creamer in tea or coffee.
- Use salmon or mackerel with bones instead of tuna in sandwiches, salads or casseroles.

- If you make your own soups add 1 or 2 tblsp. vinegar when you boil the bones for stock. The acid dissolves the calcium out of the bones, making the homemade soup as good a source of calcium as milk—and you'll never taste the vinegar.

IRON

FOOD SOURCES OF IRON

	MEAT/ ALTERNATES	VEGETABLE/ FRUIT	GRAIN
Good Sources:	pates liverwurst liver organ meats		iron-fortified cereals
Fair Sources:	beans & peas, dried beef chicken eggs nutritional yeasts nuts turkey sardines seeds shrimp	apricots, dried broccoli greens peaches, dried prune juice prunes raisin spinach squash, winter tomato juice watermelon	bread, whole grain cereals, whole grain oatmeal rice tortillas, corn or flour wheat germ

Remember: Your body's uptake of iron is improved when you combine iron sources with vitamin C foods or animal products.

VITAMIN C

FOOD SOURCES OF VITAMIN C

Good Sources:	asparagus bell pepper broccoli brussels sprouts cabbage cantaloupe cauliflower grapefruit grapefruit juice green chili	orange orange juice salsa potato strawberries spinach tomato tomato juice turnip

To Increase Iron:
- Choose vitamin C rich foods with your meals; this improves your body's uptake of iron.
- Try meat, fish, and poultry to get more iron from other foods eaten.
- Cook foods in cast iron cookware to add iron to your diet.
- Reduce the amount of tea and coffee you drink with meals as these beverages reduce the amount of iron you get from food.

SNACKS

THIRSTY!
cold milk
mineral water with
 a lime squeeze!
fruit juice
 apple
 grape
 grapefruit
 orange
 pineapple
 raspberry
chilled vegetable
 juice
lemon water
fruit juice and
 tonic or mineral
 water

JUICY!
fresh fruit
 fruit leather
 berries
 cantaloupe
 grapes
 grapefruit
 kiwi
 nectarine
 orange
 peach
 pear
 pineapple
 plum
 tangerine
 tomato
 watermelon
 frozen juice pops

SMOOTH!
yogurt
banana
papaya
mango
custard
cottage cheese
Fruit Smoothie*

FUN!
frozen grapes
dried fruit
frozen banana
fruit leather

CRUNCH!
raw veggies
 asparagus
 bell pepper
 broccoli
 cabbage
 carrots
 cauliflower
 cucumber
 jicama
 zucchini
apple
corn on the cob
puffed rice cakes
wheat crackers

REALLY HUNGRY!
hard cooked egg
apricot
granola
leftovers
sandwich
cereal with milk
bran muffin
nuts
cheese
seeds
pizza
peanut butter on
 bread, or
 crackers or
 celery

*Fruit Smoothie Recipe: Blend one cup of skim milk, 3 ice cubes, your favorite fresh or frozen fruit (ours are peaches and bananas), a dash of vanilla, cinnamon, and nutmeg in blender. Presto! A refreshing, ever pleasing sensation!

The preceding nutritional information was initially developed and written for the Health and Environment Department, State of New Mexico.

APPENDIX E

WEEKLY GOAL SHEETS
ACTIVITY JOURNAL/LOG

WEEK ONE

Because I care about my whole self, I will commit myself to the following this week:

1. I will be aerobically active _____ times.
2. The activities I have chosen are _____ .
3. I will keep track of the times I am active and my feelings before and after my activity. I will describe their kind and intensity. I will note thoughts which I have while I am active and afterwards.

THIS IS MY SPECIAL WAY OF APPRECIATING MY BODY THIS WEEK.

_____
(SIGNATURE)

WEEK TWO

Because I care about my whole self, I will commit myself to the following this week:

1. I will be aerobically active _____ times.
2. The activities I have chosen are _____ .
3. I will keep track of the times I am active and my feelings before and after my activity. I will describe their kind and intensity. I will take notice of thoughts I have during my active time.

THIS IS MY WAY OF BECOMING MORE FIT THIS WEEK.

_____
(SIGNATURE)

WEEK THREE

Because I care about my whole self, I will commit myself to the following this week:

1. I will be aerobically active _____ times.

2. The activities I have chosen are _____ .

3. I will keep track of the times I am active and my feelings before and after my activity. I will describe their kind and intensity. I will note thoughts which I have while I am active and afterwards.

THIS IS MY SPECIAL WAY OF EXPERIENCING CHANGE THIS WEEK.

_____
(SIGNATURE)

WEEK FOUR

Because I care about my whole self, I will commit myself to the following this week:

1. I will be aerobically active _____ times.

2. The activities I have chosen are _____ .

3. I will keep track of the times I am active and my feelings before and after my activity. I will describe their kind and intensity. I will take notice of thoughts I have during my active time.

THIS IS MY WAY OF GROWING STRONGER THIS WEEK.

_____
(SIGNATURE)

WEEK FIVE

Because I care about my whole self, I will commit myself to the following this week:

1. I will be aerobically active _____ times.

2. The activities I have chosen are _____ .

3. I will keep track of the times I am active and my feelings before and after my activity. I will describe their kind and intensity. I will note thoughts which I have while I am active and afterwards.

THIS IS MY SPECIAL WAY OF BEING IN TOUCH WITH MY BODY THIS WEEK.

_____
(SIGNATURE)

WEEK SIX

Because I care about my whole self, I will commit myself to the following this week:

1. I will be aerobically active _____ times.

2. The activities I have chosen are _____ .

3. I will keep track of the times I am active and my feelings before and after my activity. I will describe their kind and intensity. I will take notice of thoughts I have during my active time.

THIS IS MY WAY OF CELEBRATING LIFE THIS WEEK.

_____
(SIGNATURE)

WEEK SEVEN

Because I care about my whole self, I will commit myself to the following this week:

1. I will be aerobically active _____ times.

2. The activities I have chosen are _____ .

3. I will keep track of the times I am active and my feelings before and after my activity. I will describe their kind and intensity. I will note thoughts which I have while I am active and afterwards.

THIS IS MY SPECIAL WAY OF BECOMING AN ATHLETIC WOMAN THIS WEEK.

_____

(SIGNATURE)

WEEK EIGHT

Because I care about my whole self, I will commit myself to the following this week:

1. I will be aerobically active _____ times.

2. The activities I have chosen are _____ .

3. I will keep track of the times I am active and my feelings before and after my activity. I will describe their kind and intensity. I will take notice of thoughts I have during my active time.

THIS IS MY WAY OF BEING ME THIS WEEK.

_____

(SIGNATURE)

JOURNAL/LOG

Type (i.e. run)	Intensity (10-second heart rate)	How Long?	Feelings & Thoughts

Monday

Tuesday

Wednesday

Thursday

Friday

Saturday

Sunday

(COPY THIS SHEET AND USE WEEKLY ... USE THE BACK TOO!)

APPENDIX F

RELAXATION TECHNIQUES

HINTS ON HOW TO RELAX
Relaxing a Tense Body:

By Breathing: Inhale through your nose slowly, hold, and exhale through your mouth slowly. Take about five counts to inhale, five counts to hold and five counts to exhale; pause and repeat. Think only about your breathing.

By Letting Go: Close your eyes, or look down. Let your jaw slack, drop your shoulders, sigh audibly. Hold nothing in—stomach, chest, buttocks, etc.

By Shaking: Stand or sit with your arms hanging loosely; shake your hands, then your arms. Increase the vigor of your shaking, then slowly subside until you are still once more. Feel the quiet. Repeat.

By Imagery: Breathe slowly. Quiet your thoughts. Create an image in your mind's eye of a lovely place which you know. Get a clear sense of how it looks, sounds, smells, feels, etc. Be there. Be refreshed by its power and its restful quality. Choose to end the image, knowing that you can return to it again.

By Prayer: Breathe in slowly; exhale slowly. As you breathe in say to yourself, "God lives," as you exhale, say, "in me now." Or choose any meaningful phrase or mantra, i.e., "Shalom," "Peace," or simply, "One," or "Om."

HOW TO BRING FORTH THE
RELAXATION RESPONSE
Adapted From *The Relaxation Response* **Herbert Benson**

Go to a quiet place where you can be alone and undisturbed.
Choose a mental device (phrase or image upon which to focus).
Have a passive attitude.
Assume a comfortable position.

—Sit quietly in this comfortable position.

—Close your eyes.

—Deeply relax all of your muscles, one by one, beginning at your feet and progressing up to your face. Mentally tell them it is all right to let go of tension; it is all right to relax.

—Breathe through your nose; pay attention to your breathing, the sound of it, the feel of it.

—As you breathe out say the word, "one" silently to yourself. Breathe easily and slowly. Don't strain or think about "trying to do this right," just breath and say the word "one."

—Continue doing this for 10 to 20 minutes. You may open your eyes to check the time, but don't use any alarms which interrupt and jolt you.

—If a distraction comes, gently move it aside. Remind yourself that you are relaxing, not thinking of any thing right now.

(You might try this daily, even twice a day—or only a few times a week. You decide. It is for you. It is for life.)

A QUICK CALMING POSTURE

Designed to last about 15 seconds (could be longer if you wish). To be used when things are chaotic and you want to grab a moment for yourself.

• Discriminate an annoying stimulant. (For example, the telephone, a particular voice, excessive noise, pressure to perform well.)
• Smile (inside, or outside) and say to yourself: "Leave my body out of this."
• Take two deep breaths. Take about 4 to 6 counts for this.
• As you exhale the second breath, relax your jaw and let the relaxed feeling spread from your jaw to your neck, shoulders, back, arms, hands, chest, abdomen, hips, thighs, calves, ankles, feet, toes.
• Resume your activities. (Perhaps, a bit more slowly.)

INDEX

Processed foods, 81
Pulse, finding, 27-28

R

Racquet sports, 25
Radial pulse, 27-28
Realistic, being and motivation, 128-29
Relaxation Response, The (Benson), 91, 169
Relaxation techniques, 169-70
Religious beliefs, and body image, 109-119
Rest, 43
Restrictive eating, 67
R.I.C.E. formula, 43-44
Rohé, Fred, 85, 113, 114
Roller skating, 25
Rope skipping, 147
Rothfarb, Ruth, 125
Runners "high," 13-14
Running, 25, 114, 139-40. *See also* Walking
  clothing for, 141
  equipment for, 140-41
  tips for, 141

S

Saccharin, 77
Safflower oil, 80
Salt, 82
Saturated fats, 80
Scale, 66
Scott-Maxwell, Florida, 1
Seidal, Kay Morris, 123
Self-esteem, 86
  and body appearance, 12
  need for, 11-12
Self-talk, and motivation, 129
Sex, 102-6
Sexual health, and active life, 106-8
Shoes
  running/walking, 140
  walking, 138
Side and overhead stretch, 33
Side leg raises, 39
Single knee press, 36
Sit-stretch, 35

Skill building exercises, 24
Skin fold calipers, 19
Snacks, 82-83, 160
Snyder, Gary, 113
Socks, 138, 141
Sodium, 82
Softball, 24
Soft drinks, 78
Soleus stretch, 41
Solitude, and handling stress, 92
Sorbitol, 77
Soy oil, 80
Spare tire pinch, 21
Spinning, 144
  tips for, 145
Spiritual, getting, about the physical, 119-21
Spirituality
  non-denominational, 116-18
  twelve-step, 118-19
Spiritual pursuits, 120
Spiritual Wellness (Pilch), 116
Sports bras, 141, 150-51
Sprains, 43
Square dancing, 25
Stair climbing, 147
Stationary cycling program, 146
Stationary running, 147
Stewart, Gordon, W., 15
Strains, 43
Strength, 9
  increasing physical, 7
  need for inside, 7-9
Strengthening exercises, 24
Stress
  handling, 90-93
  identifying sources of, 87-90
  living with, 85-93
  signs of, 86-87
Stretching, 24
Styrofoam, 143
Sugar, 82
Sunglasses, 151
Sun Protection Factor (SPF), 151
Sunscreen, 58, 151
Supplements, 83
Sweat band, 58, 145
Swimming, 2, 3, 25
  equipment for, 58, 142-43
  tips for, 143-44

ALSO AVAILABLE FROM PARKSIDE PUBLISHING

BOOKS:

- FREEDOM FROM FOOD. Through six case histories, told with compelling immediacy in the first person, author Elizabeth Hampshire develops a careful picture of addiction and its treatment. Order #6449 $8.95

- GROWING THROUGH THE PAIN: The Incest Survivor's Companion. Exploring Incest as it is experienced, from the inside, this book brings companionship, hope, validation, and inspiration to the incest survivor. Order #6750 $9.95

- HELP FOR HELPERS: Daily Meditations for Counselors. This collection of 366 daily readings was written by counselors from all over the country. Order #6725 $6.95

- SIBS: The Forgotten Family Members. Written by Nancy Hull-Mast and Diane Purcell, this book emerged from a therapy group for the siblings of addicted adolescents, the "forgotten" family members whose own emotional lives have been put on hold and who have now begun to recognize and nurture healthy and self-caring behaviors. Order #6760 $6.95

- TOMORROW, MONDAY, OR NEW YEAR'S DAY: Emerging Issues in Eating Disorder Recovery. Joan Ebbitt, MSW, outlines the conflicts that may emerge in recovery, steps to deal with these issues, and the many rewards of recovery from an eating illness. Order #6748 $6.95

PAMPHLETS:

- TALKING TO A HIGHER POWER, by Catherine H. A collection of inspiring stories, many people speak of their journey toward and contact with a Higher Power. An important re-introduction to spirituality for anyone in recovery. Order #6752 $1.50

- HONESTY. Defining *honesty* as "existing when our behavior is consistent with our inner selves," this booklet of exercises helps young people in early recovery prepare for a good Fourth Step. Written by Nancy Hull-Mast. Order #6757 $1.25

To order call:
1-800-221-6364
In Illinois call 312-698-8550
(For Illinois residents: After Nov. 11, 1989, our new phone number will be
708-698-8550
